Foot Bones Anatomy

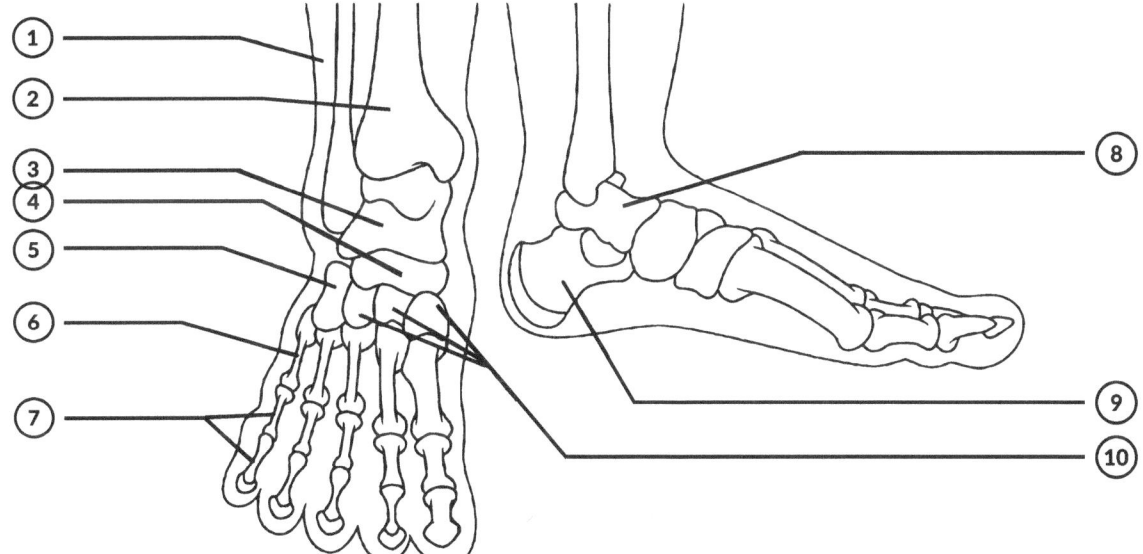

Foot Bones Anatomy

(1). Fibula
(2). Tibia
(3). Talus(Ankle Bone)
(4). Navicular
(5). Cuboid
(6). Metatarsals
(7). Phalanges
(8). Talus(Ankle Bone)
(9). Calcaneus (Heel Bone)
(10). Cuneiforms

THIS BOOK BELONGS TO

_____

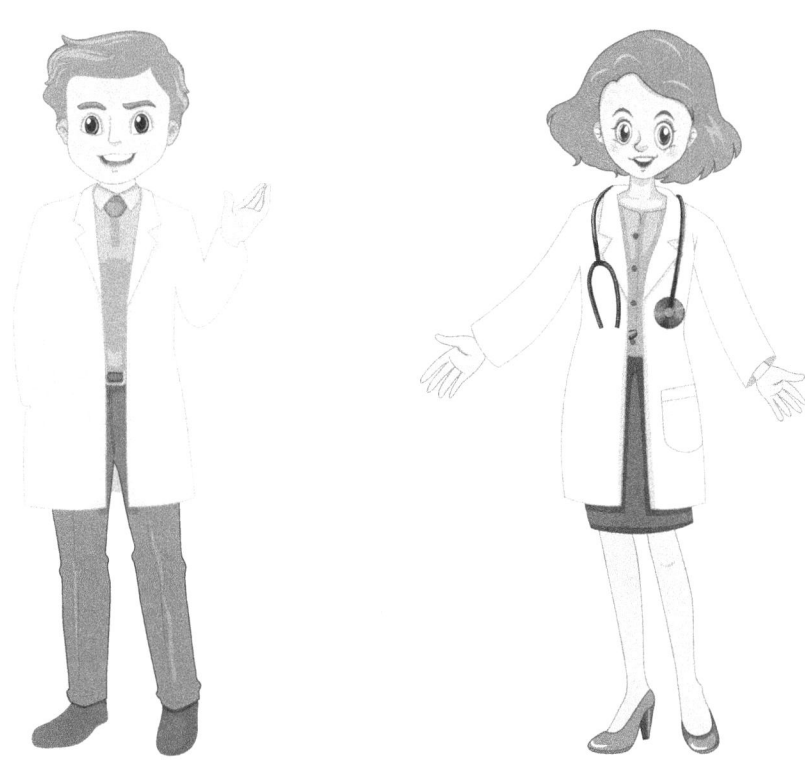

Brain Anatomy

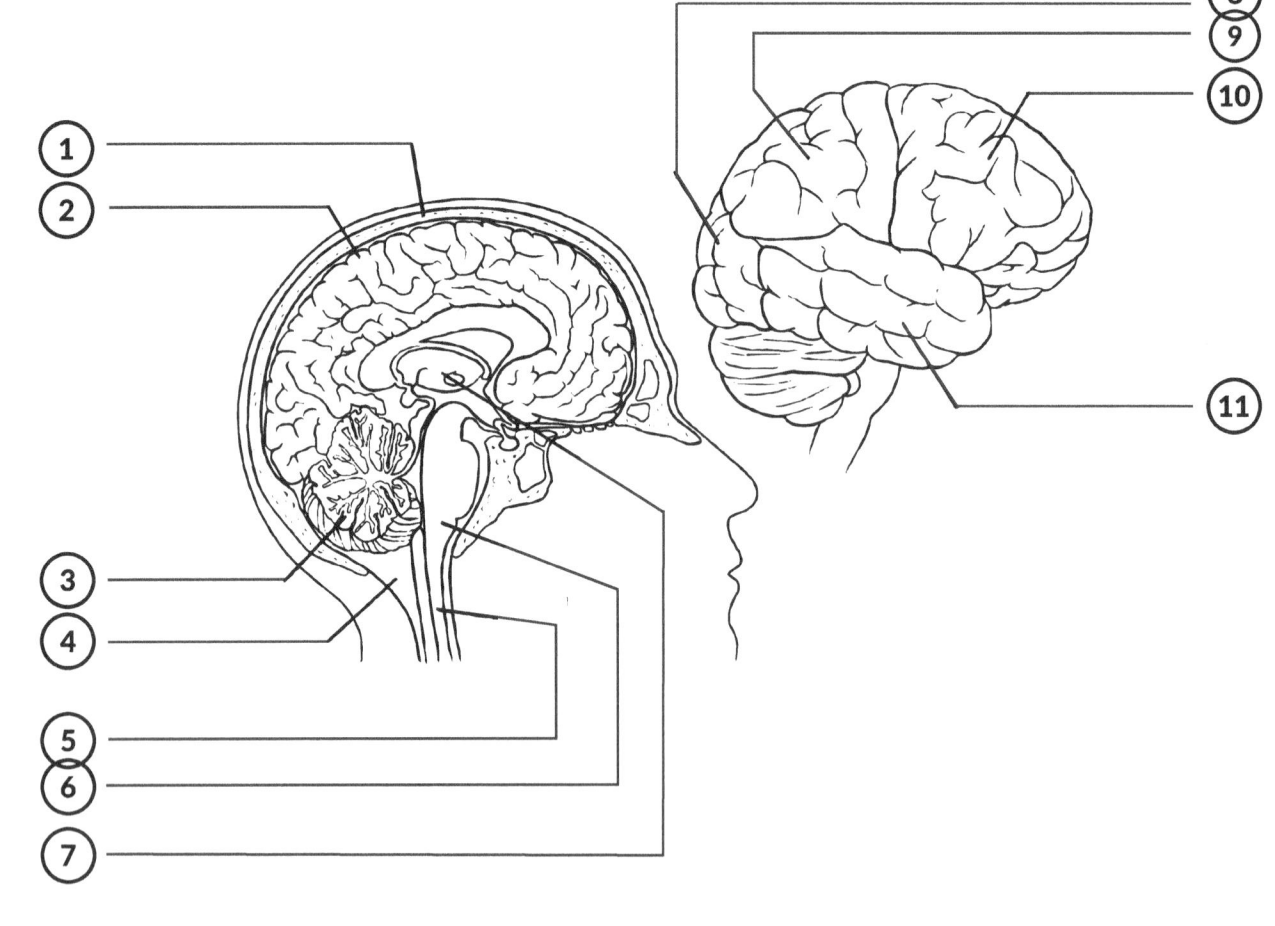

Brain Anatomy

(1). Cranium
(2). Corex
(3). Cerebellum
(4). Dura
(5). Spinal Cord
(6). Brain Stem
(7). Basal Ganglia
(8). Occipital Lobe
(9). Parietal Lobe
(10). Frontal Lobe
(11). Temporal Lobe

Eye Anatomy

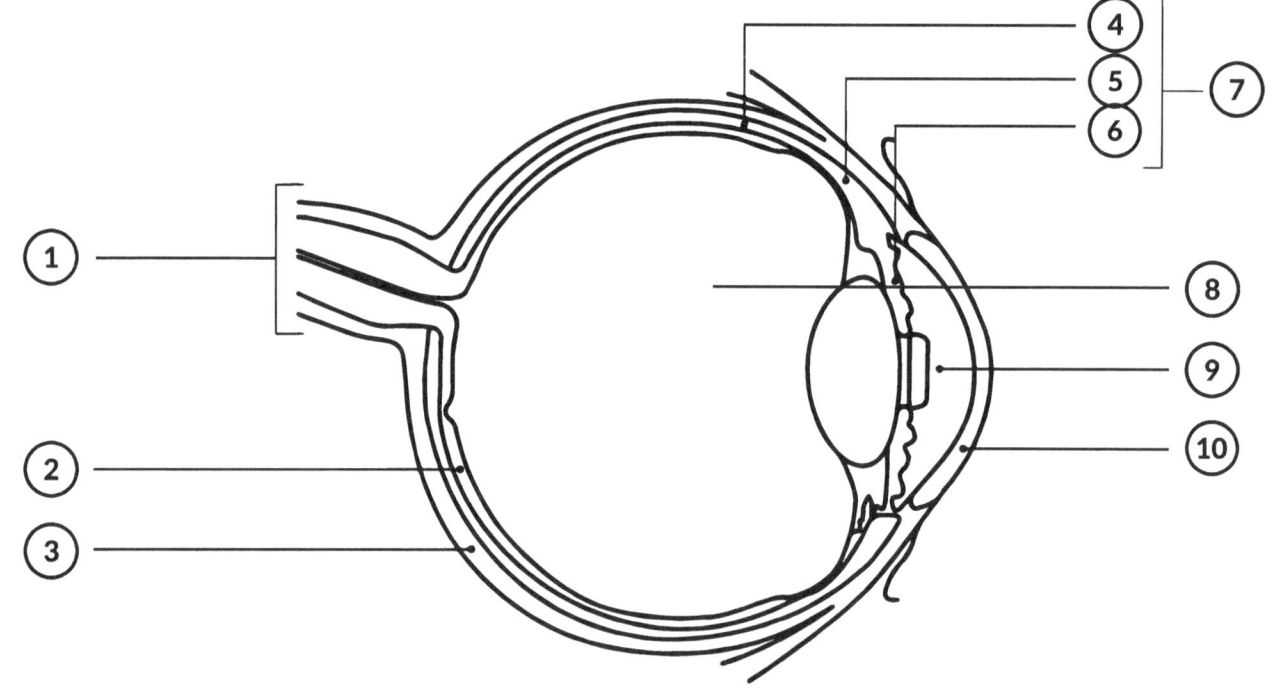

Eye Anatomy

(1). Optic Nerve

(2). Retina

(3). Sclera

(4). Choroid

(5). Ciliary Body

(6). Iris

(7). Uvea

(8). Vitreous

(9). Pupil

(10). Cornea

Tongue Anatomy

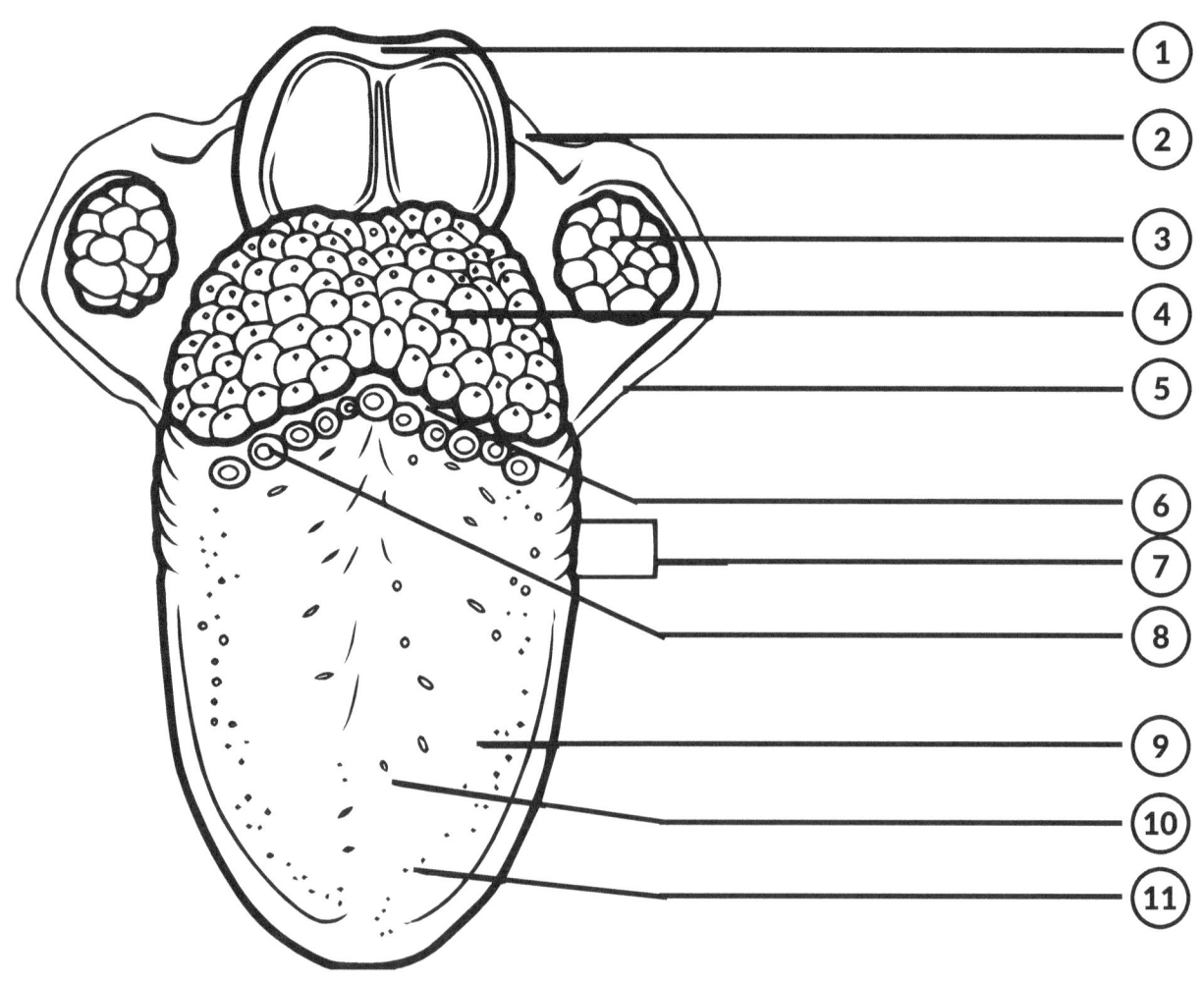

Tongue Anatomy

(1). Epiglottis
(2). Palatopharyngeal Arch
(3). Palatine Tonsil
(4). Lingual Tonsil
(5). Palatoglossal Arch
(6). Terminal Sulcus
(7). Foliate Papillae
(8). Circumvallate Papilla
(9). Dorsum Of Tongue
(10). Fungiform Papilla
(11). Filiform Papilla

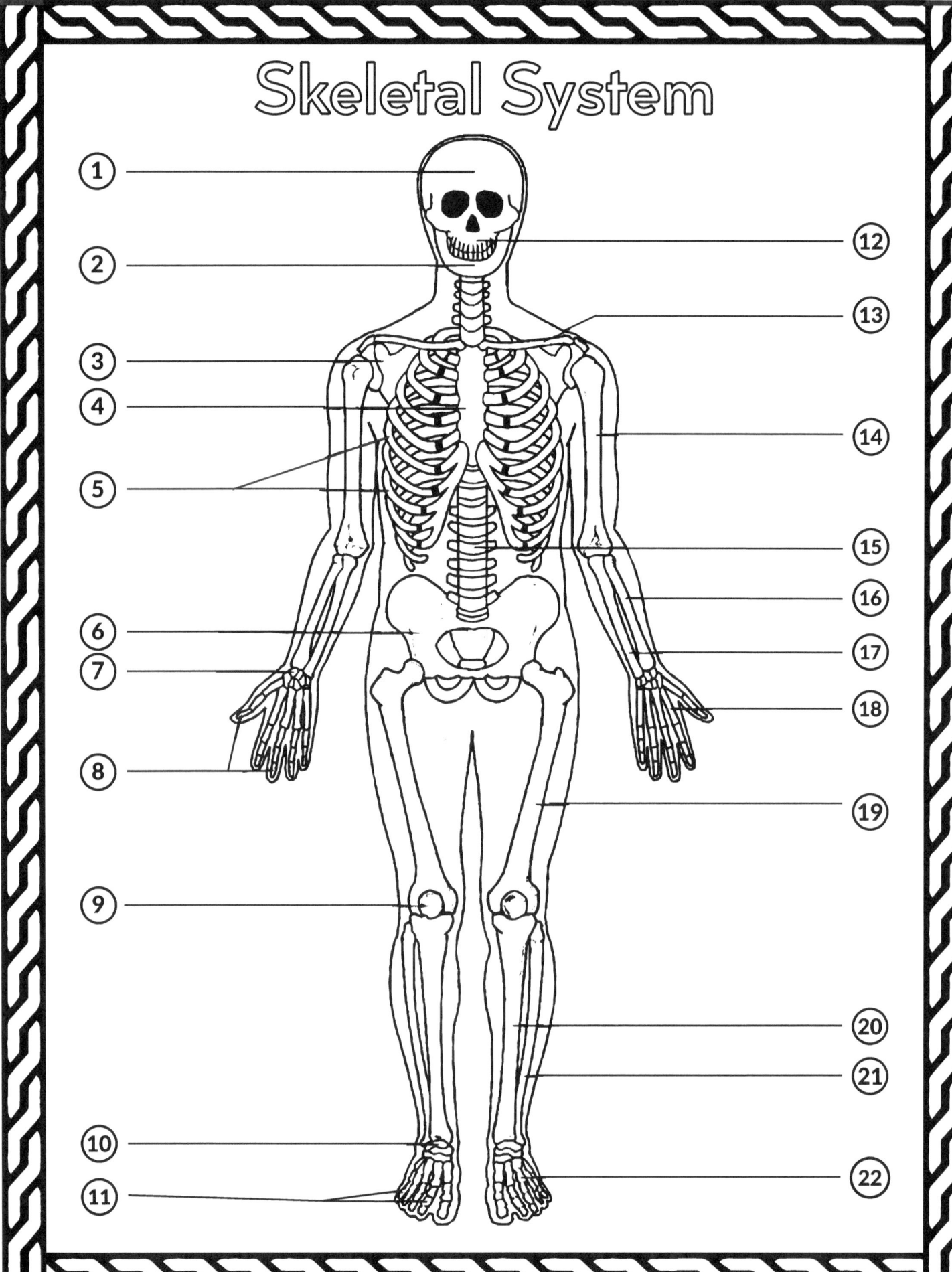

Skeletal System

(1). Cranium
(2). Mandible
(3). Scapula
(4). Sternum
(5). Ribs
(6). Pelvis
(7). Carpals
(8). Phalanges
(9). Patella
(10). Tarsals
(11). Phalanges
(12). Maxilla
(13). Clavicle
(14). Humerus
(15). Vertebral Column
(16). Radius
(17). Ulna
(18). Metacarpals
(19). Femur
(20). Tibia
(21). Fibula
(22). Metatarsals

Urinary System

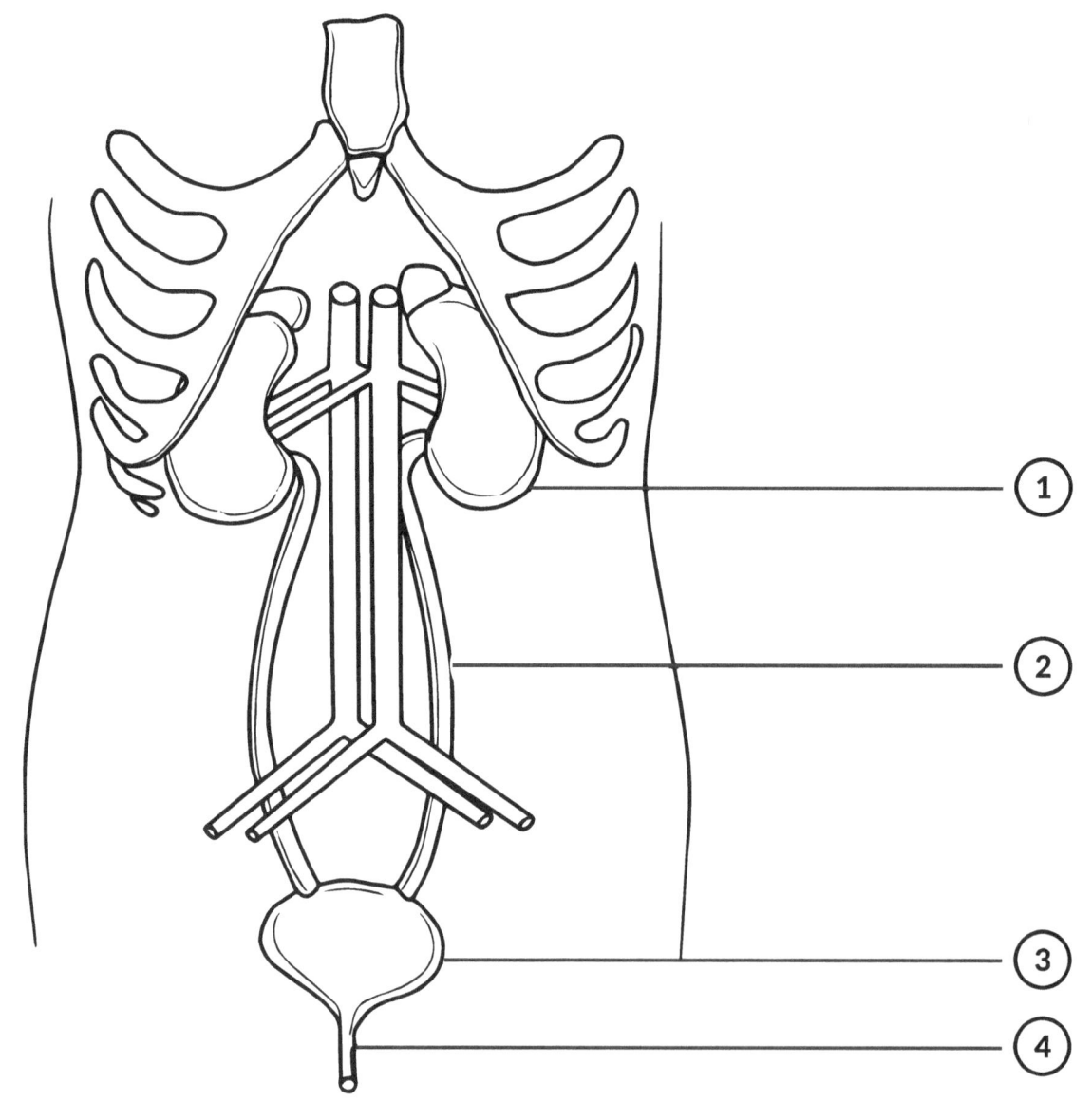

1.
2.
3.
4.

Urinary System
(1). Kidney

(2). Ureter

(3). Bladder

(4). Urethra

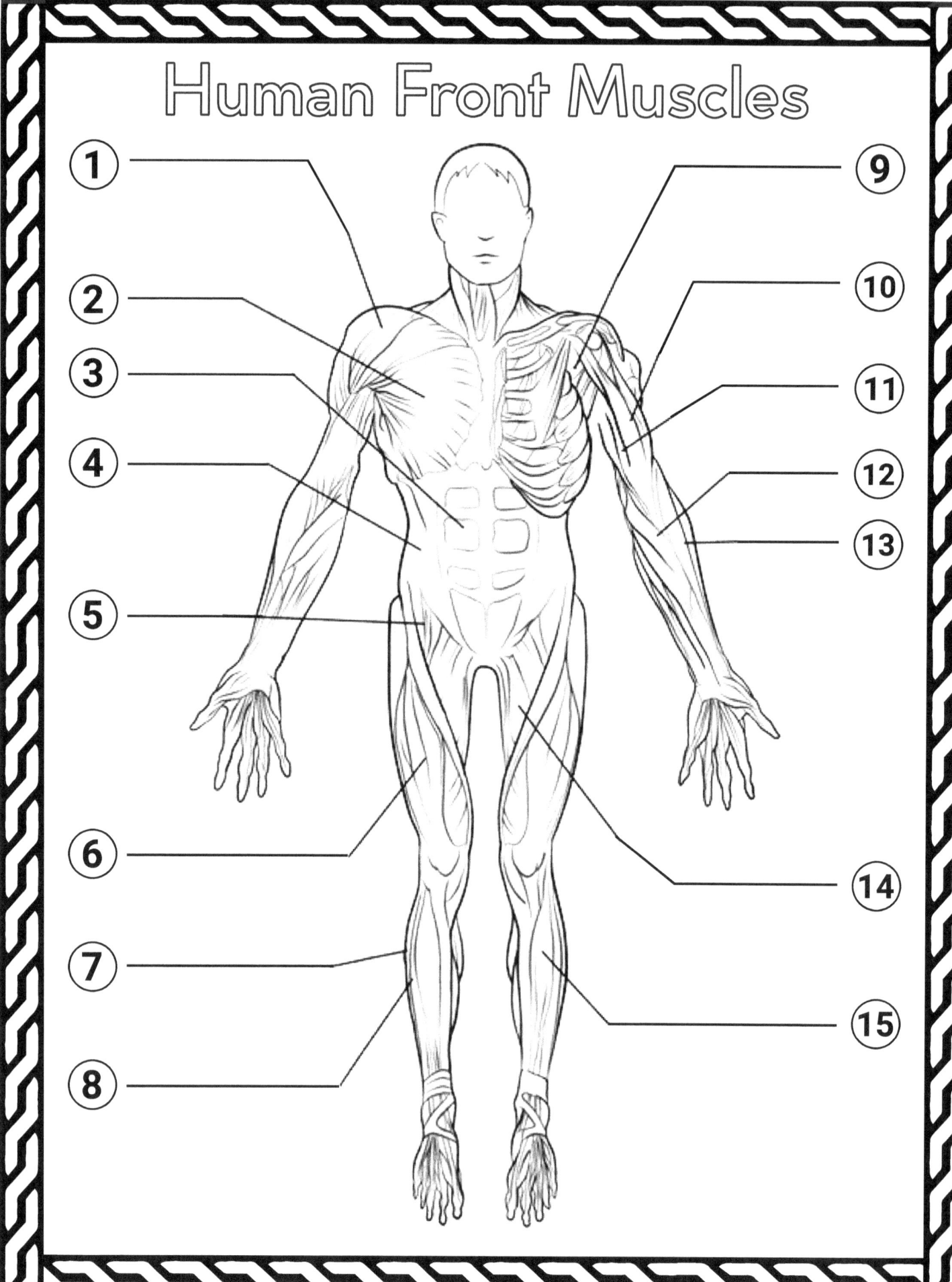

Human Front Muscles

(1). Deltoid
(2). Pectoralis Major
(3). Rectus Abdominis
(4). Abdominal External Oblique
(5). Iliopsoas
(6). Quadriceps Femoris
(7). Peroneus Longus
(8). Peroneus Brevis
(9). Rotator Cuff
(10). Biceps Brachii
(11). Brachialis
(12). Pronator Teres
(13). Brachioradialis
(14). Adductor Muscles
(15). Tibialis Anterior

Heart Anatomy

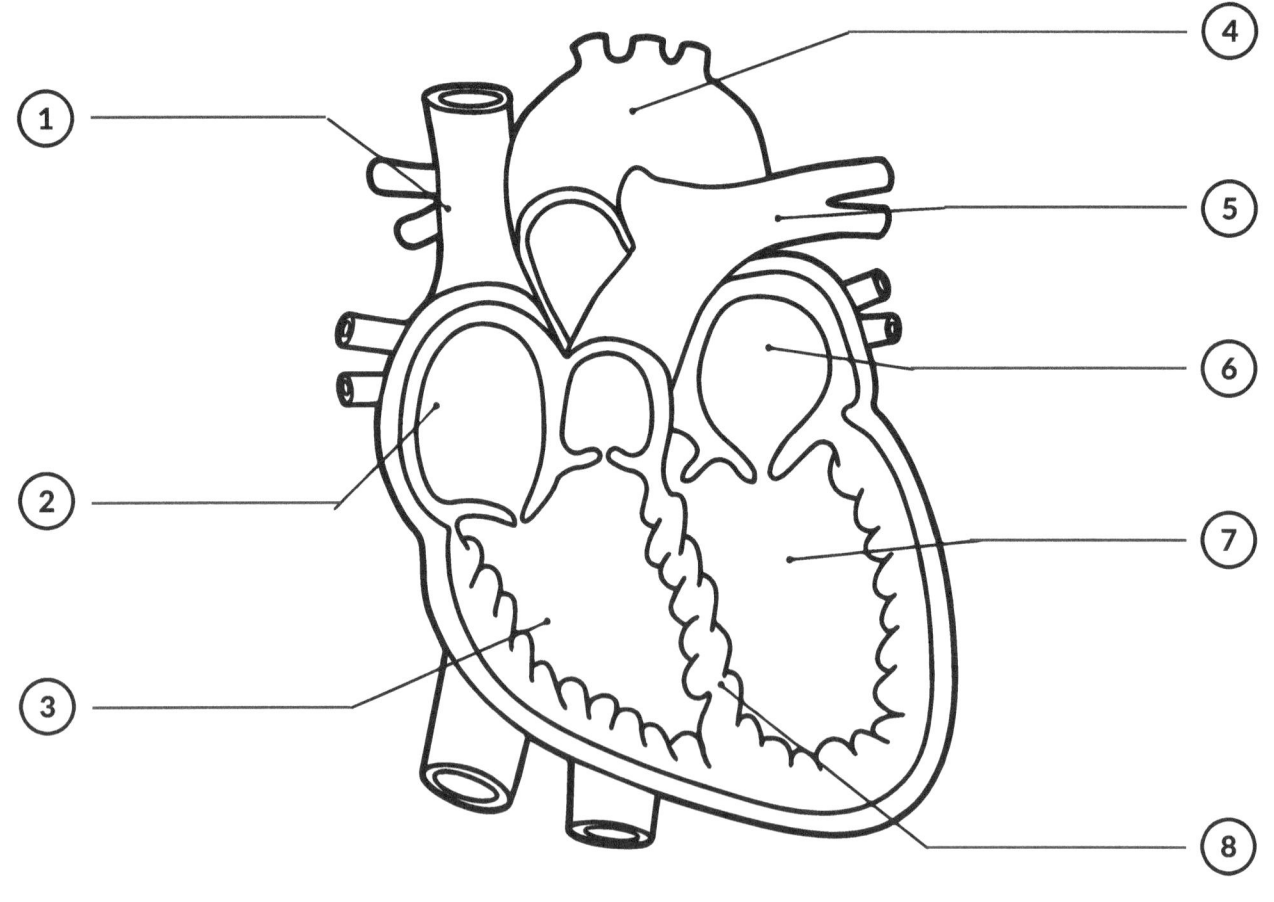

Heart Anatomy

(1). Superior Vena Cava
(2). Right Atrium
(3). Right Ventricle
(4). Aorta
(5). Pulmonary Artery
(6). Left Atrium
(7). Left Ventricle
(8). Interventricular Septum

immune system

immune system

(1). Tonsils And Adenoids
(2). Lymph Nodes
(3). Appendix
(4). Bone Marrow
(5). Lymph Nodes
(6). Lymphatic Vessels
(7). Thymus
(8). Spleen
(9). Peyer's Patches
(10). Lymph Nodes
(11). Lymphatic Vessels

Human Back Muscles

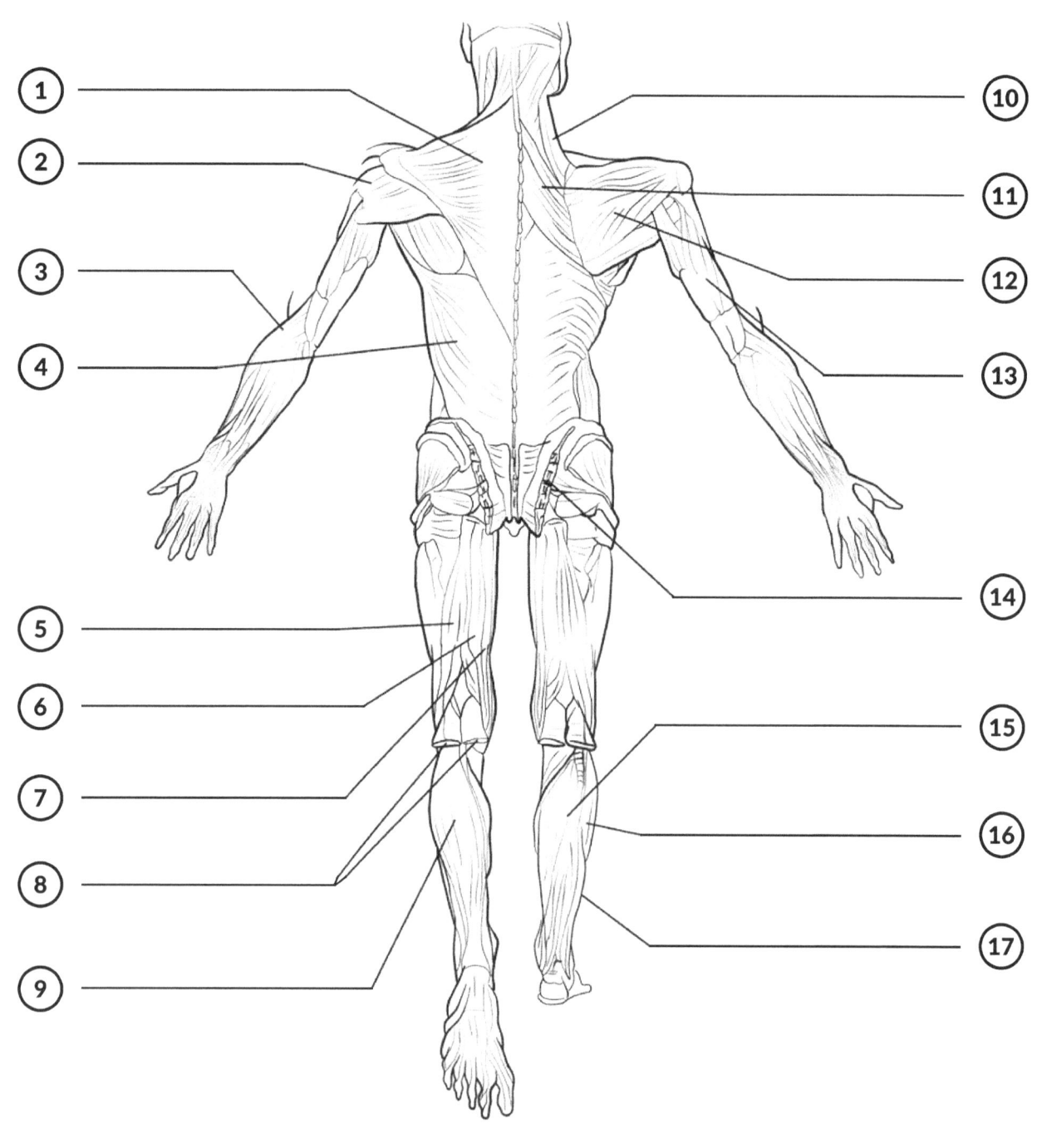

Human Back Muscles

(1). Trapezius
(2). Deltoid
(3). Brachioradialist
(4). Latissimus Dorsi
(5). Biceps Femoris
(6). Semitendinosus
(7). Semimembranosus
(8). Gastrocnemius
(9). Soleus
(10). Levator Scapulae
(11). Rhomboids
(12). Rotator Cuff
(13). Triceps Brachii
(14). Gluteus Maximus
(15). Tibialis Posterior
(16). Peroneus Longus
(17). Peroneus Brevis

Digestive System

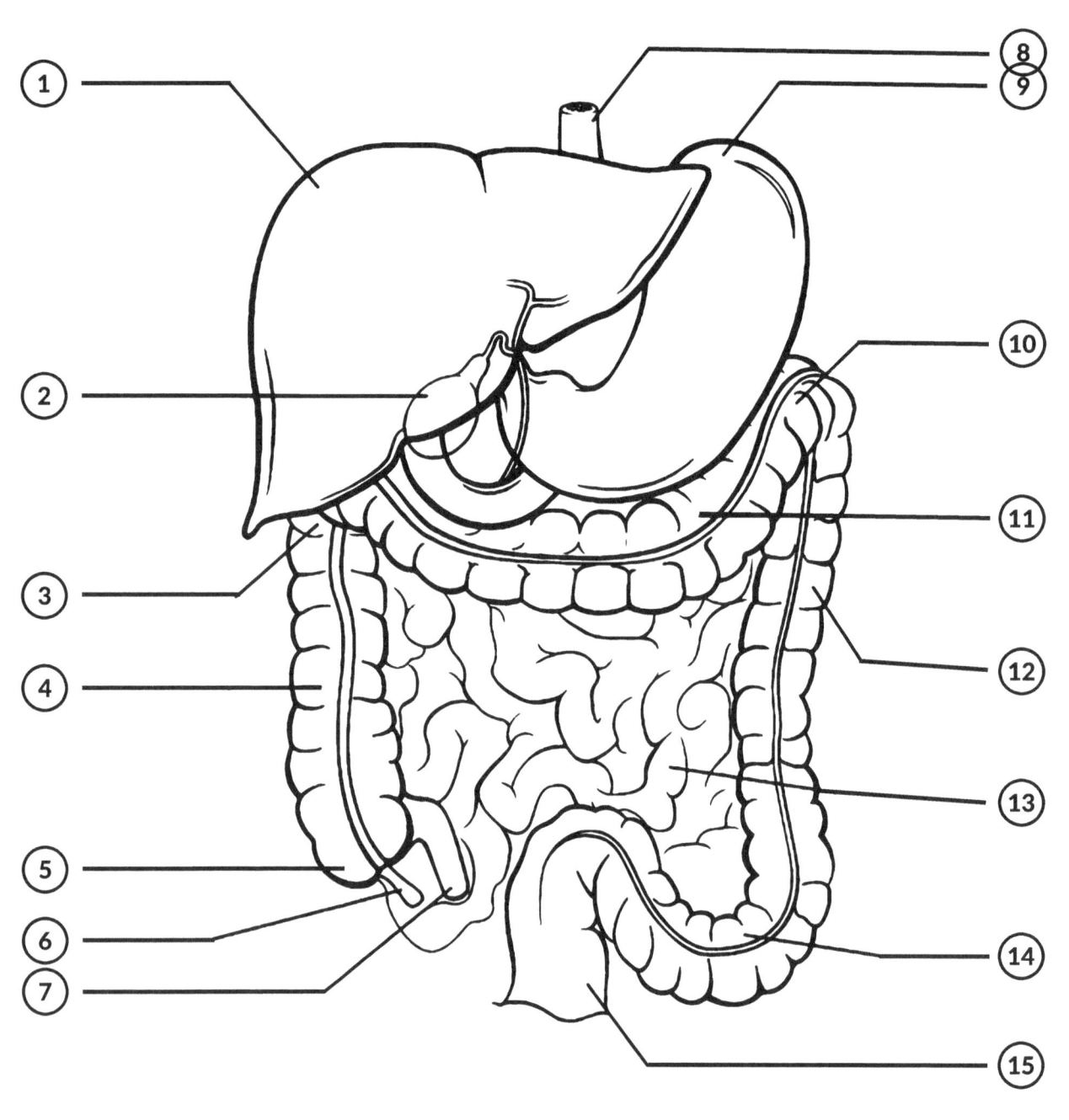

Digestive System

(1). Liver
(2). Gall Bladder
(3). Right Colic Flexure
(4). Ascending Colon
(5). Cecum
(6). Appendix
(7). Illeum
(8). Esophagus
(9). Stomach
(10). Left Colic Flexure
(11). Transverse Colon
(12). Decending Colon
(13). Small intestine
(14). Sigmoid Colon
(15). Rectum

Respiratory System

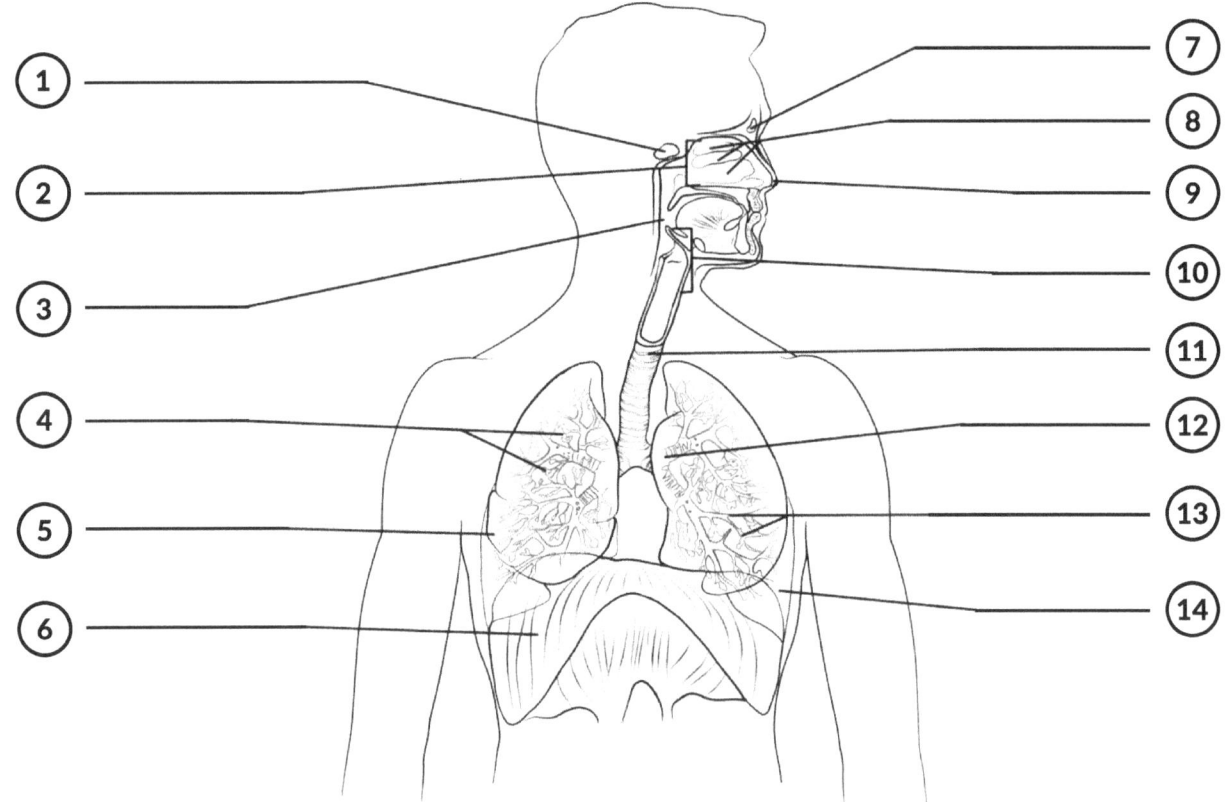

Respiratory System

(1). Sphenoidal Sinus
(2). Nasal Cavity
(3). Pharynx
(4). Alveoli
(5). Right Lung
(6). Diaphragm
(7). Frontal Sinus
(8). Nasal Conchae
(9). Nose
(10). Larynx
(11). Trachea
(12). Bronchus
(13). Bronchioles
(14). Left Lung

Kidney Anatomy

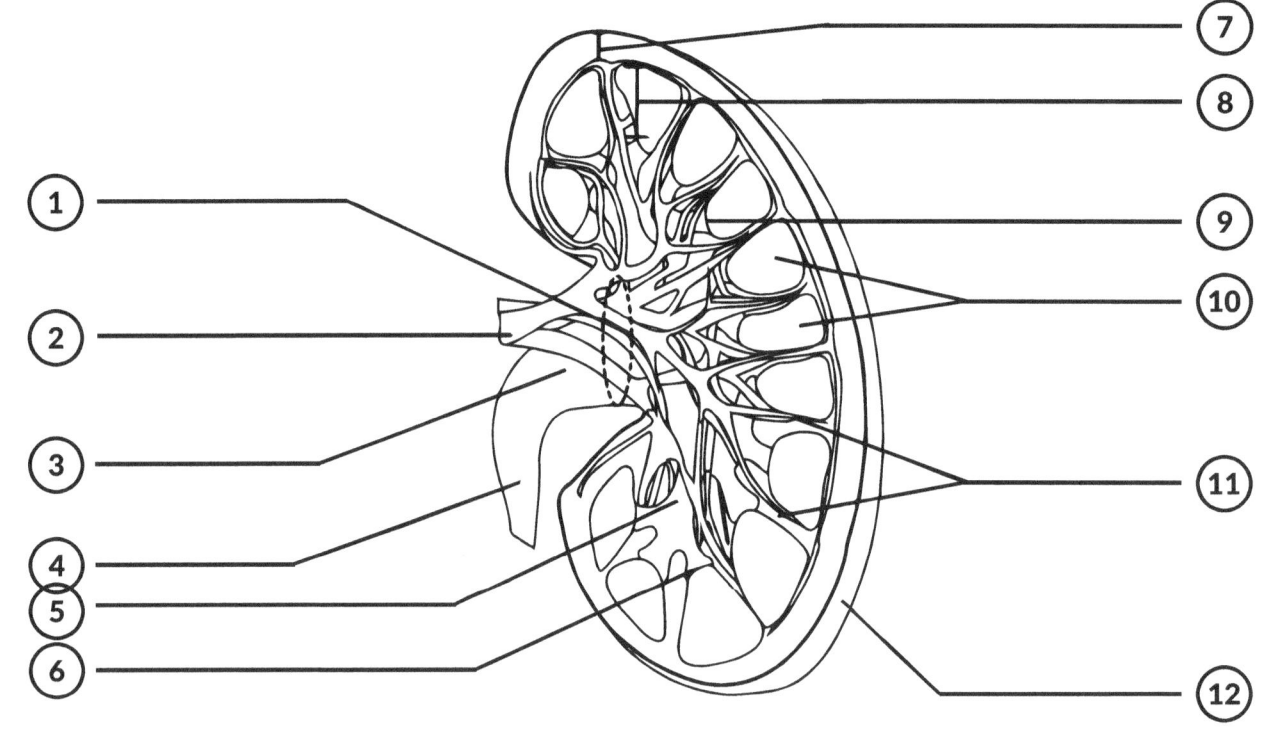

Kidney Anatomy

(1). Hilum
(2). Renal Artery Renal Vein
(3). Renal Pelvis
(4). Ureter
(5). Major Calyx
(6). Minor Calyx
(7). Renal Cortex
(8). Renal Medulla
(9). Renal Papilla
(10). Renal Pyramids
(11). Renal Columns
(12). Fibrous Capsule

Mouth Anatomy

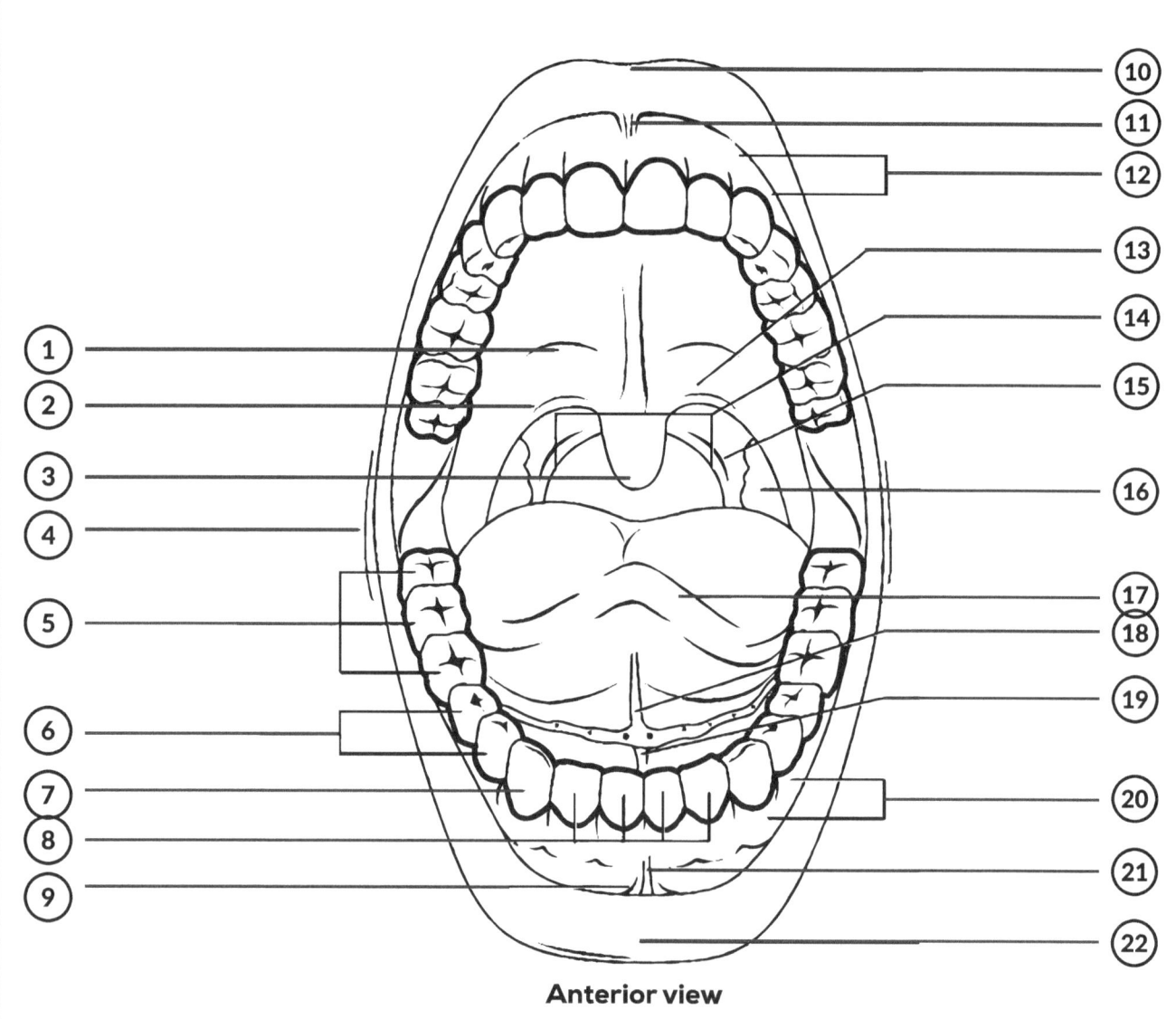

Anterior view

Mouth Anatomy

(1). Hard Palate
(2). Soft Palate
(3). Uvula
(4). Cheek
(5). Molars
(6). Premolars
(7). Cuspid (Canine)
(8). Incisors
(9). Oral Vestibule
(10). Superior Lip
(11). Superior Labial Frenulum
(12). Gingivae (Gums)
(13). Palatoglossal Arch
(14). Fauces
(15). Palatopharyngeal Arch
(16). Palatine Tonsil
(17). Tongue (Underside)
(18). Lingual Frenulum
(19). Opening Duct Of Submandibular Gland
(20). Gingivae (Gums)
(21). Inferior Labial Frenulum
(22). Inferior Lip

Skull Anatomy

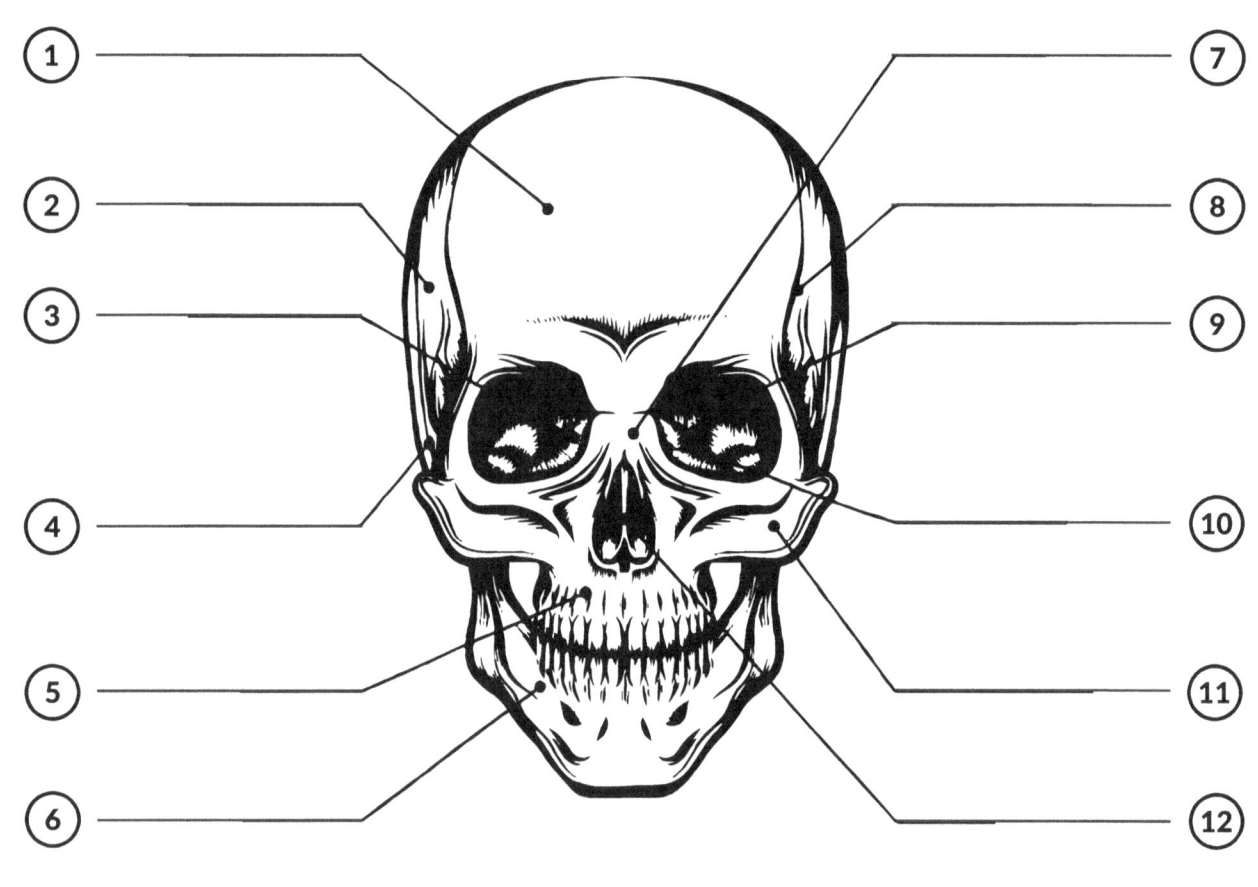

Skull Anatomy

(1). Frontal Bone
(2). Parietal Bone
(3). Ethmoid Bone
(4). Temporal Bone
(5). Maxilla
(6). Mandible
(7). Nasal Bone
(8). Coronal Suture
(9). Sphenoid Bone
(10). Lacrimal Bone
(11). Zygomatic Bone
(12). Vomer

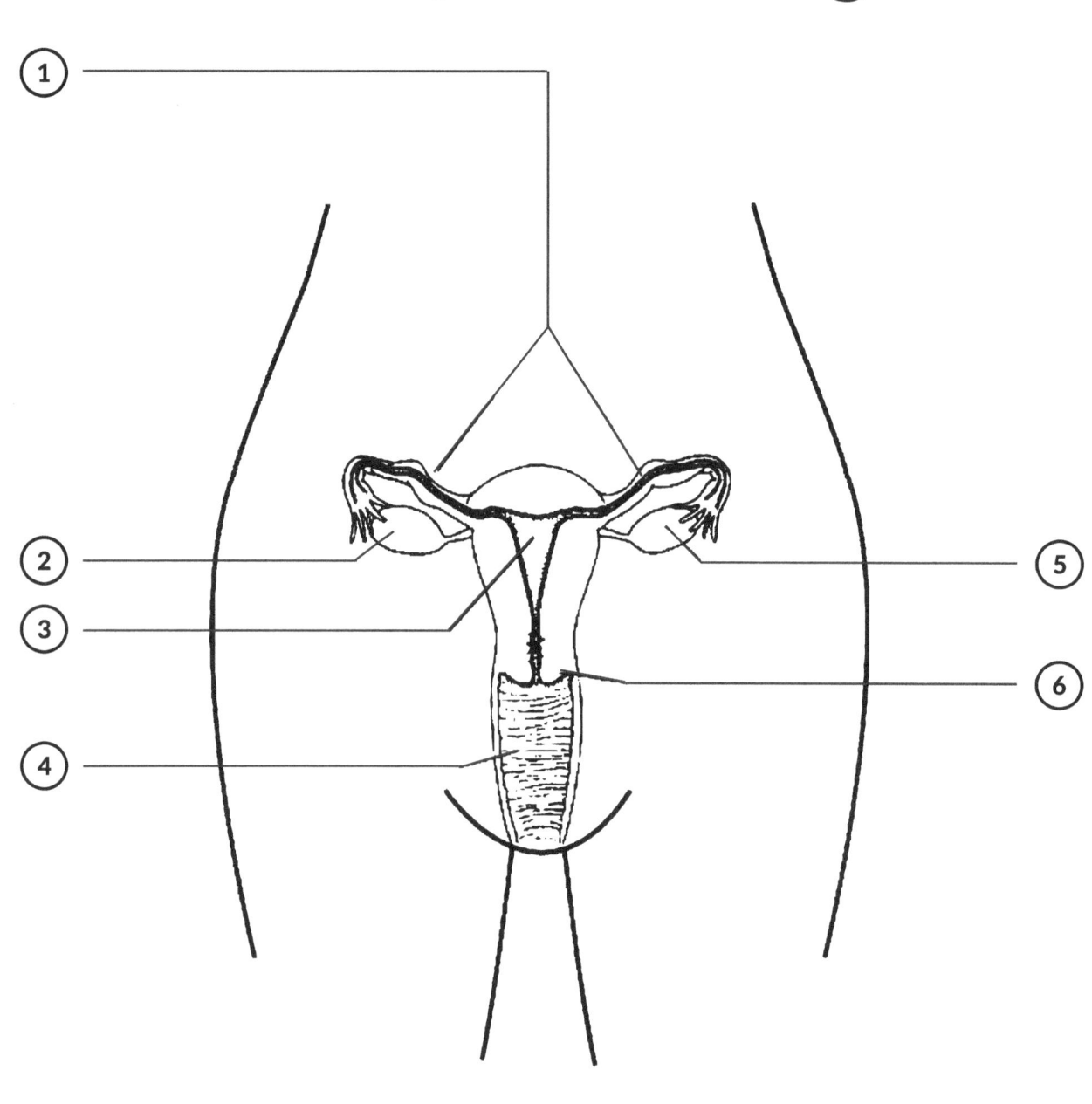

Female Reproductive Organs

(1). Fallopian Tubes
(2). Ovary
(3). Uterus
(4). Vagina
(5). Ovary
(6). Cervix

Tooth Anatomy

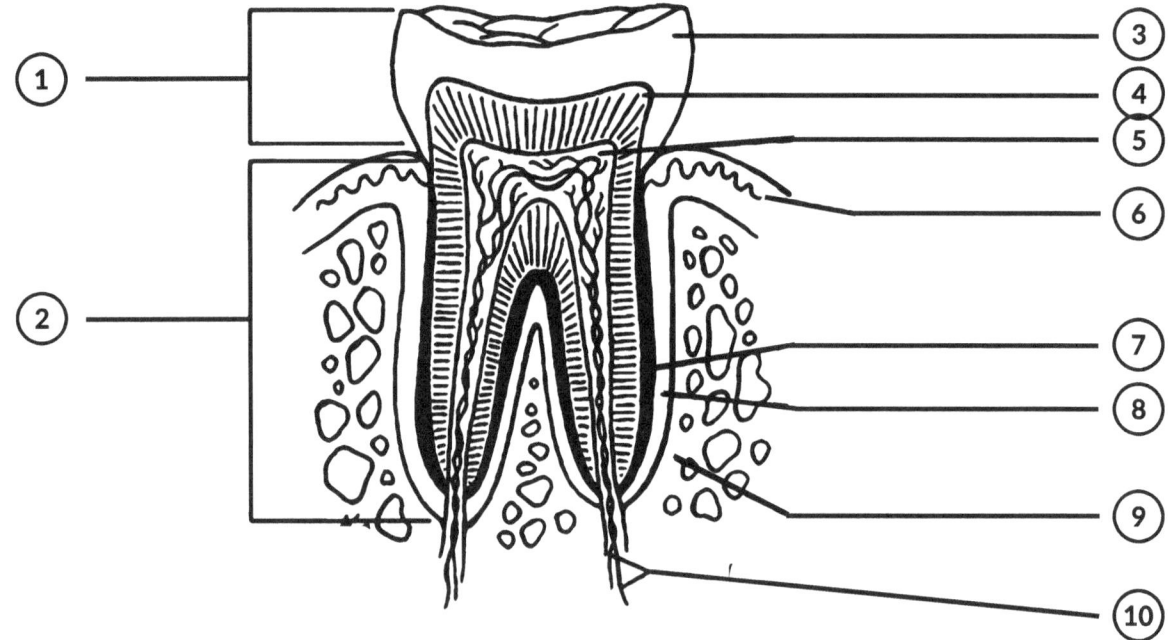

Tooth Anatomy

(1). Crown
(2). Root
(3). Enamel
(4). Dentin
(5). Pulp
(6). Gum
(7). Cementum
(8). Periodontal Membrane
(9). Bone
(10). Nerve And Blood Supply

Ear Anatomy

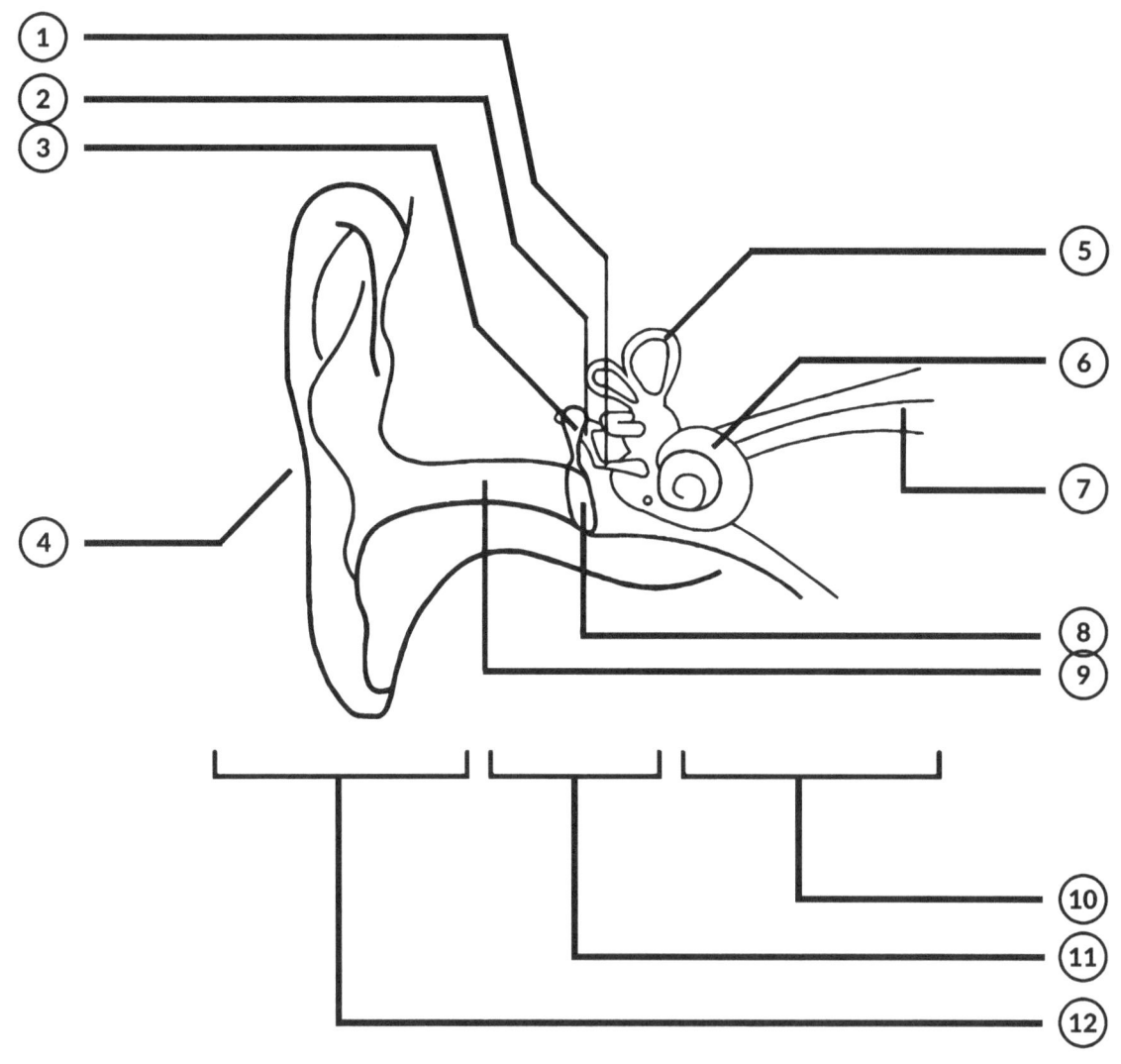

Ear Anatomy

(1). Stirrup
(2). Anvil
(3). Hammer
(4). Pinna
(5). Semicircular Canals
(6). Cochlea
(7). Auditory Nerve
(8). Ear Drum
(9). Auditory Canal
(10). Inner Ear
(11). Middle Ear
(12). Outer Ear

Endocrine System

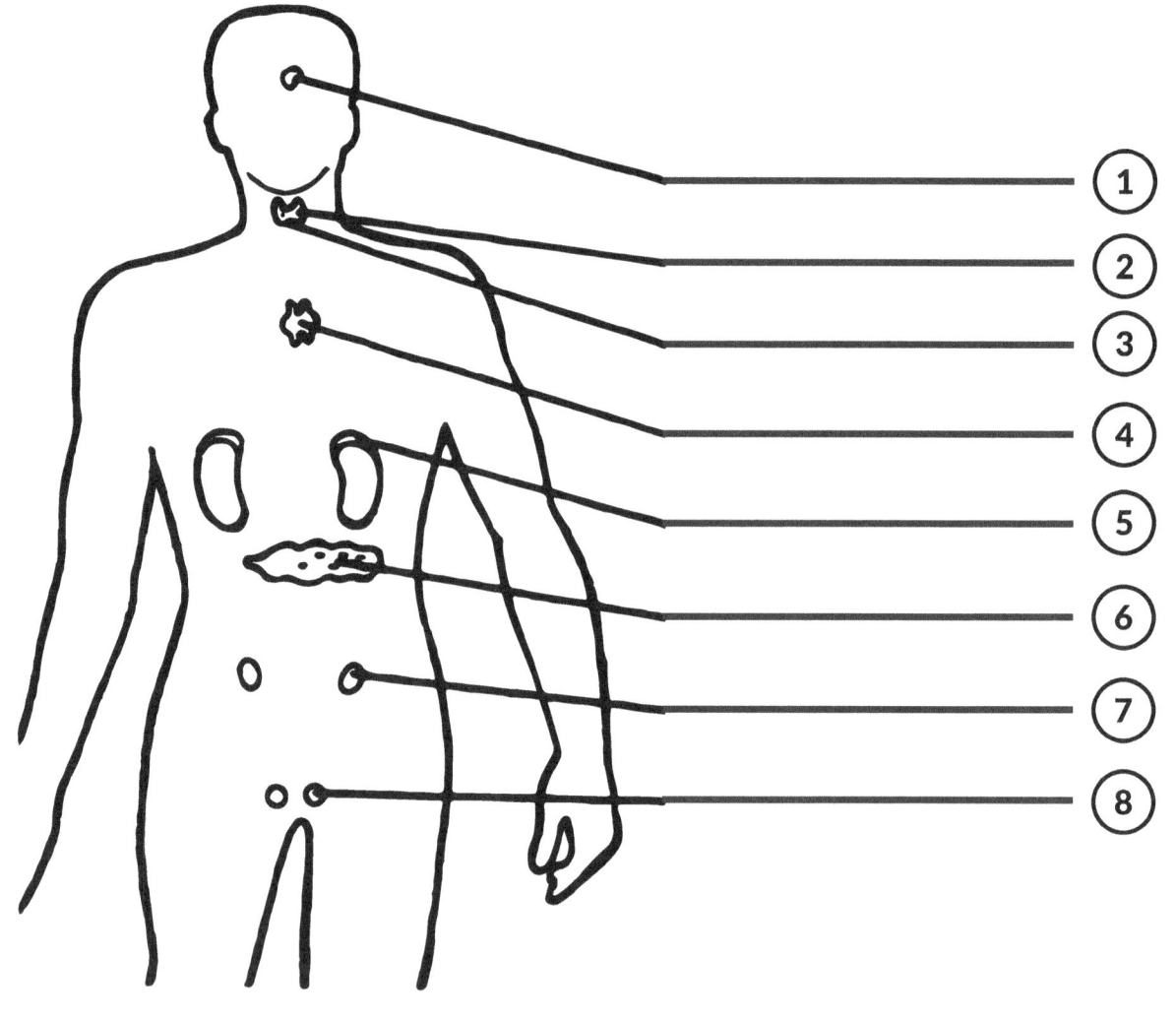

1.
2.
3.
4.
5.
6.
7.
8.

Endocrine System

(1). Pituitary Gland
(2). Parathyroid Glands
(3). Thyroid Gland
(4). Thymus Gland
(5). Adrenal Glands
(6). Island Of Langerhans
(7). Ovaries (Female)
(8). Testes (Male)

Central Nervous System

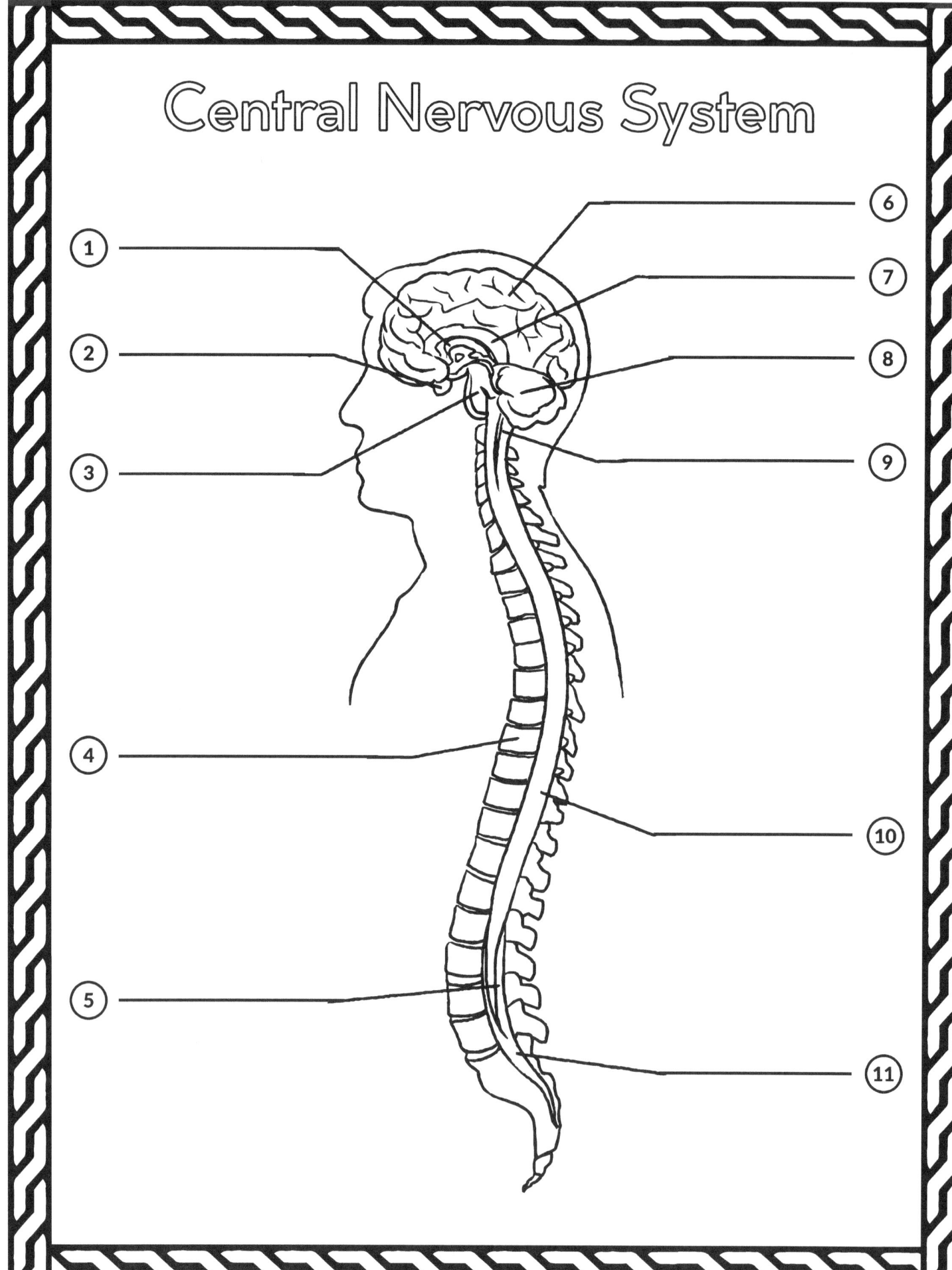

Central Nervous System

(1). Body Of Fornix
(2). Pituitary Gland
(3). Pons Varolii
(4). Vertebral Column
(5). Cauda Equina
(6). Cerebrum
(7). Corpus Callosum
(8). Cerebellum
(9). Brain Stem
(10). Spinal Cord
(11). Dura Mater

Hand Anatomy

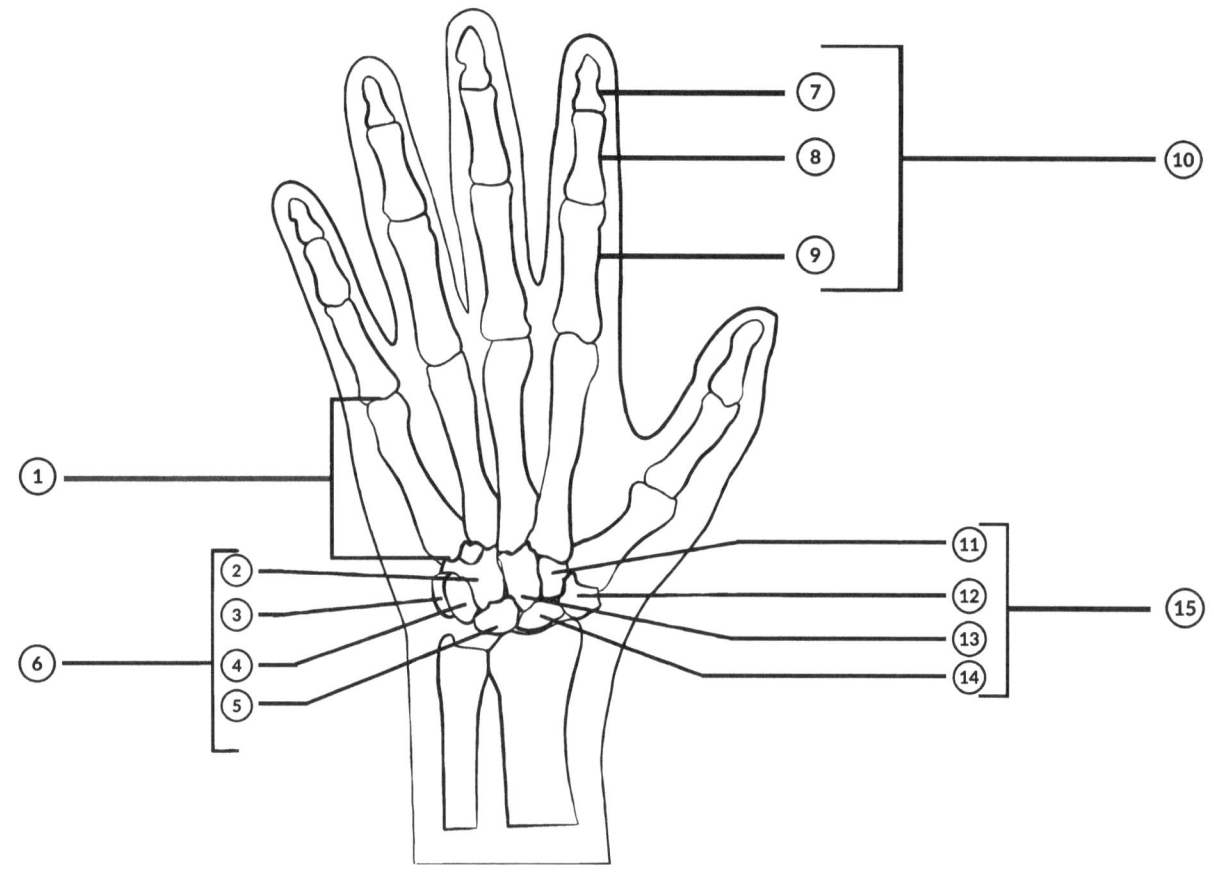

Hand Anatomy

(1). Metacarpal Bones
(2). Hamate
(3). Triquetrum
(4). Pisiform
(5). Lunate
(6). Carpal Bones
(7). Distal
(8). Middle
(9). Proximal
(10). Phalanges
(11). Trapezoid
(12). Trapezium
(13). Capitate
(14). Scaphoid
(15). Carpal Bones

Leg Anatomy

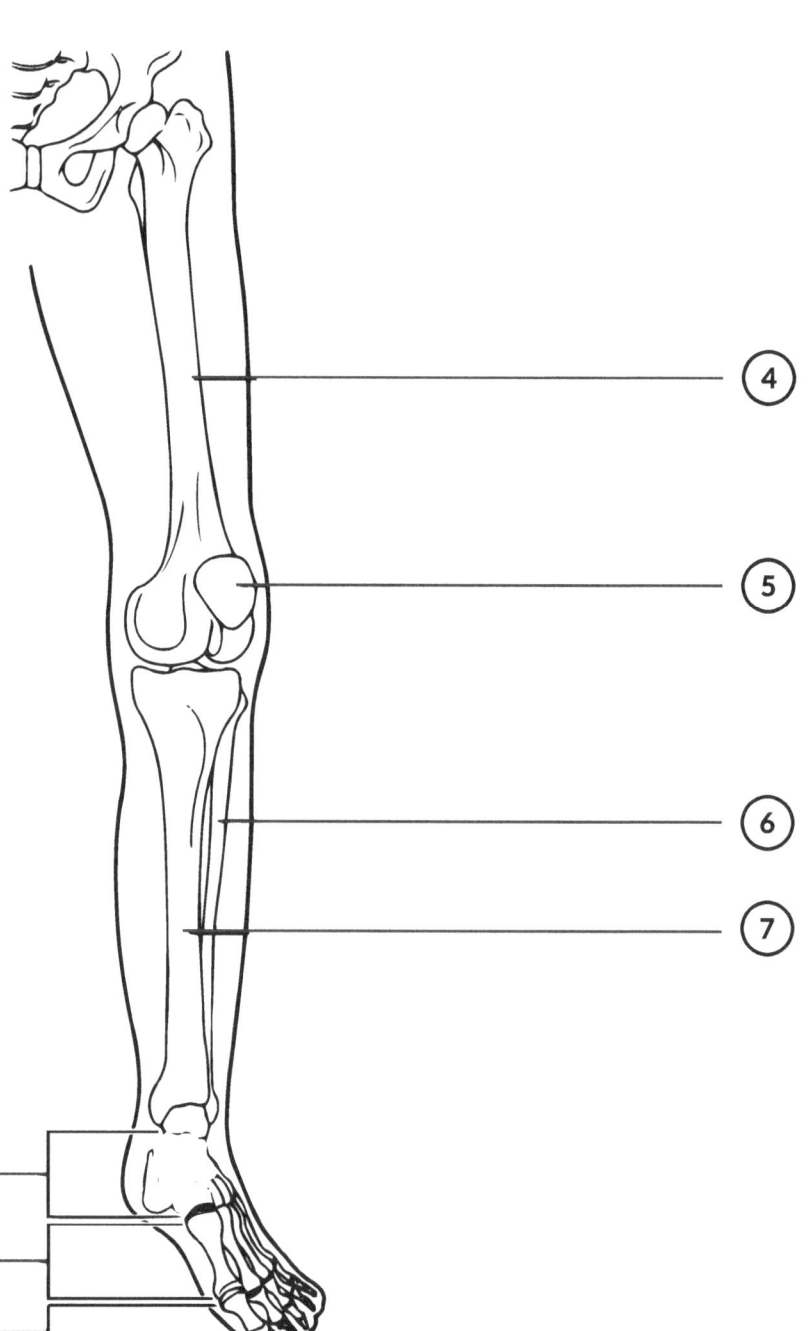

Leg Anatomy

(1). Tarsals

(2). Metatarsals

(3). Phalanges

(4). Femur

(5). Patella

(6). Fibula

(7). Tibia

Female Reproductive System

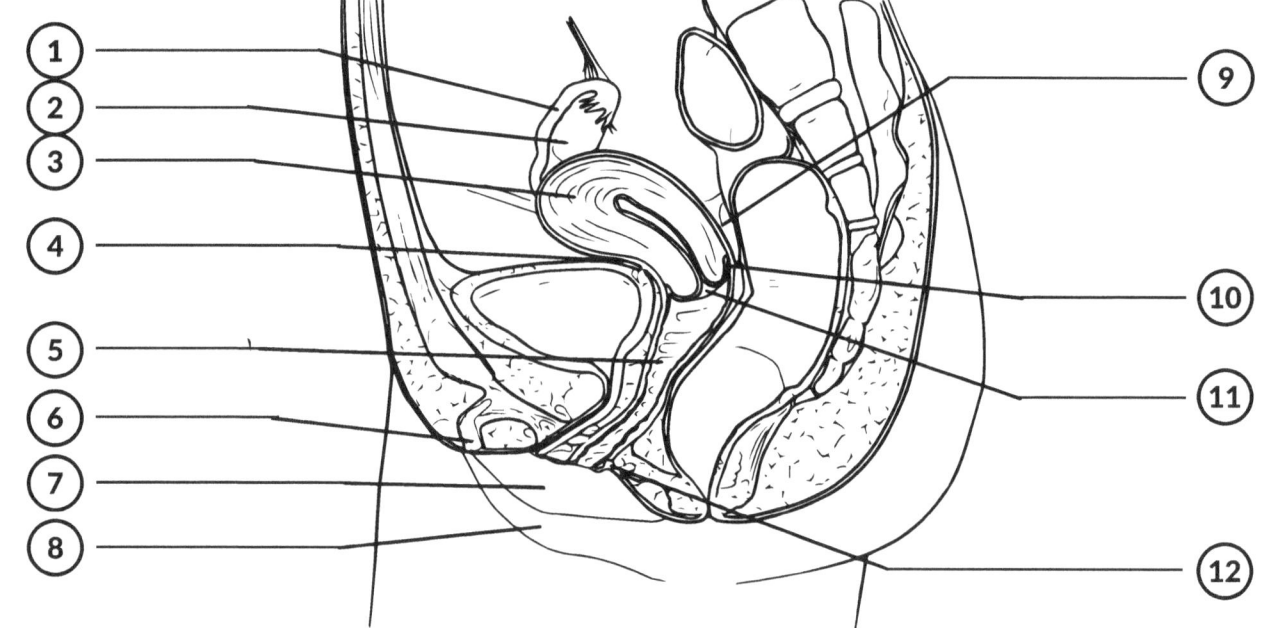

Female Reproductive System

(1). Uterine Tube
(2). Ovary
(3). Uterus
(4). Vesicouterine Pouch
(5). Vagine
(6). Clitorus
(7). Labium Minus
(8). Labium Majus
(9). Rectouterine Pouch
(10). Formix
(11). Cervix
(12). Greater Vestibular Gland

Male Reproductive System

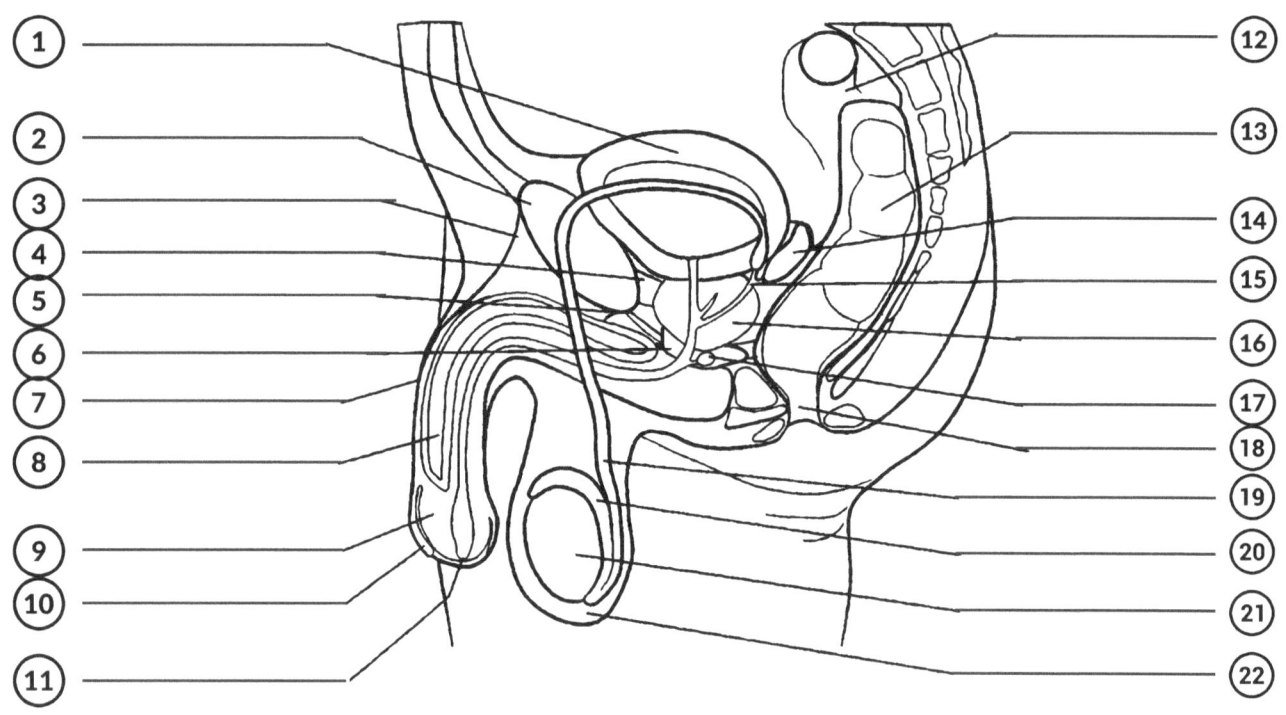

Male Reproductive System

(1). Bladder
(2). Pubic Bone
(3). Suspensory Ligament Of Penis
(4). Puboprostatic Ligament
(5). Perineal Membrane
(6). External Urethral Sphincter
(7). Penis
(8). Corpus Cavernosum
(9). Glands Penis
(10). Foreskin
(11). Urethral Opening
(12). Sigmoid Colon
(13). Rectum
(14). Seminal Vesicle
(15). Ejaculatory Duct
(16). Prostate Gland
(17). Cowper's Gland
(18). Anus
(19). Vas Deferens
(20). Epididymis
(21). Testis
(22). Scrotum

Human Body Diagram

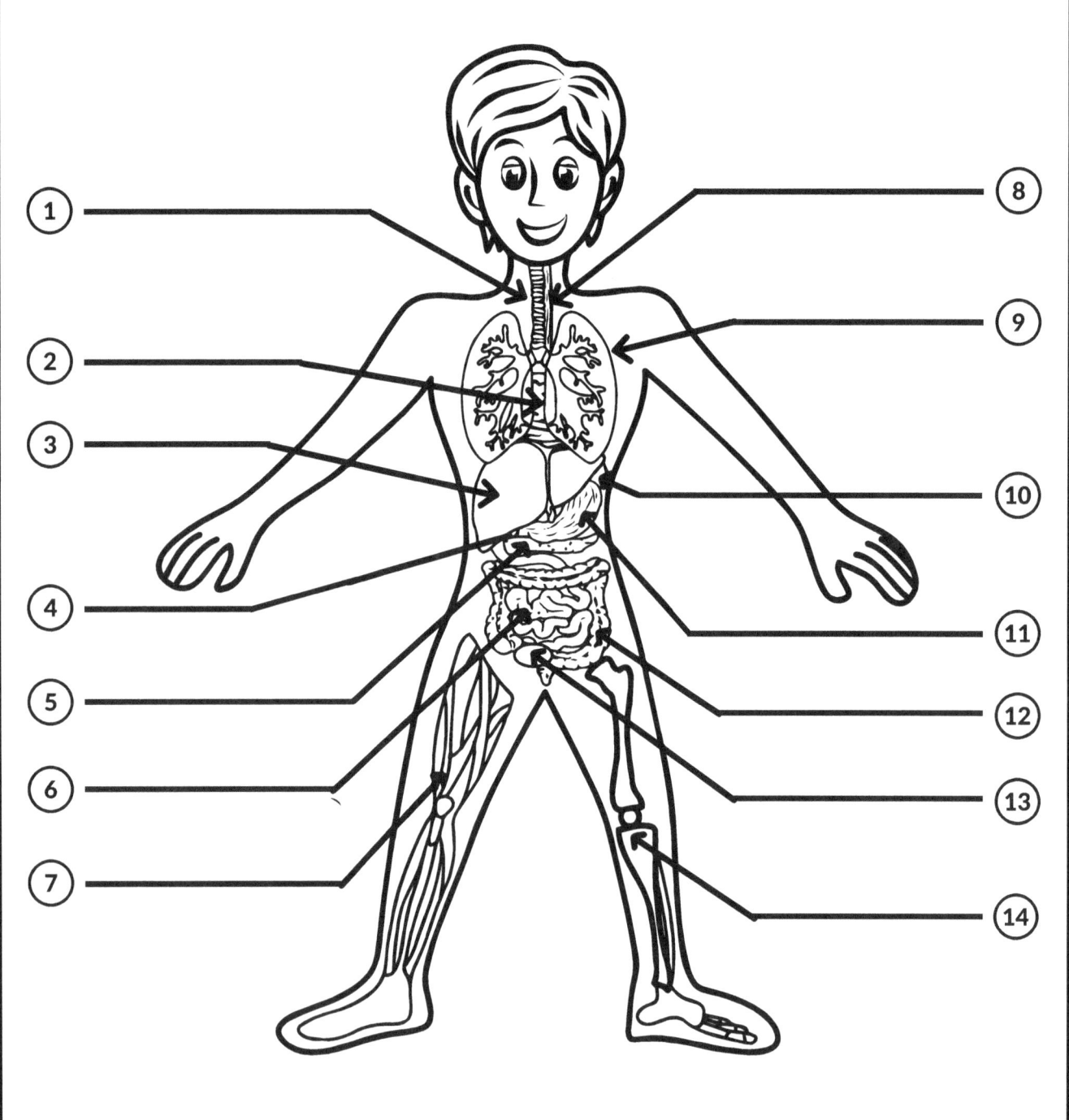

Human Body Diagram

(1). Trachea
(2). Heart
(3). Liver
(4). Gall Bladder
(5). Pancreas
(6). Small Intestine
(7). Muscle
(8). Esophagus
(9). Lungs
(10). Spleen
(11). Stomach
(12). Large Intestine
(13). Bladder
(14). Bone

Liver Anatomy

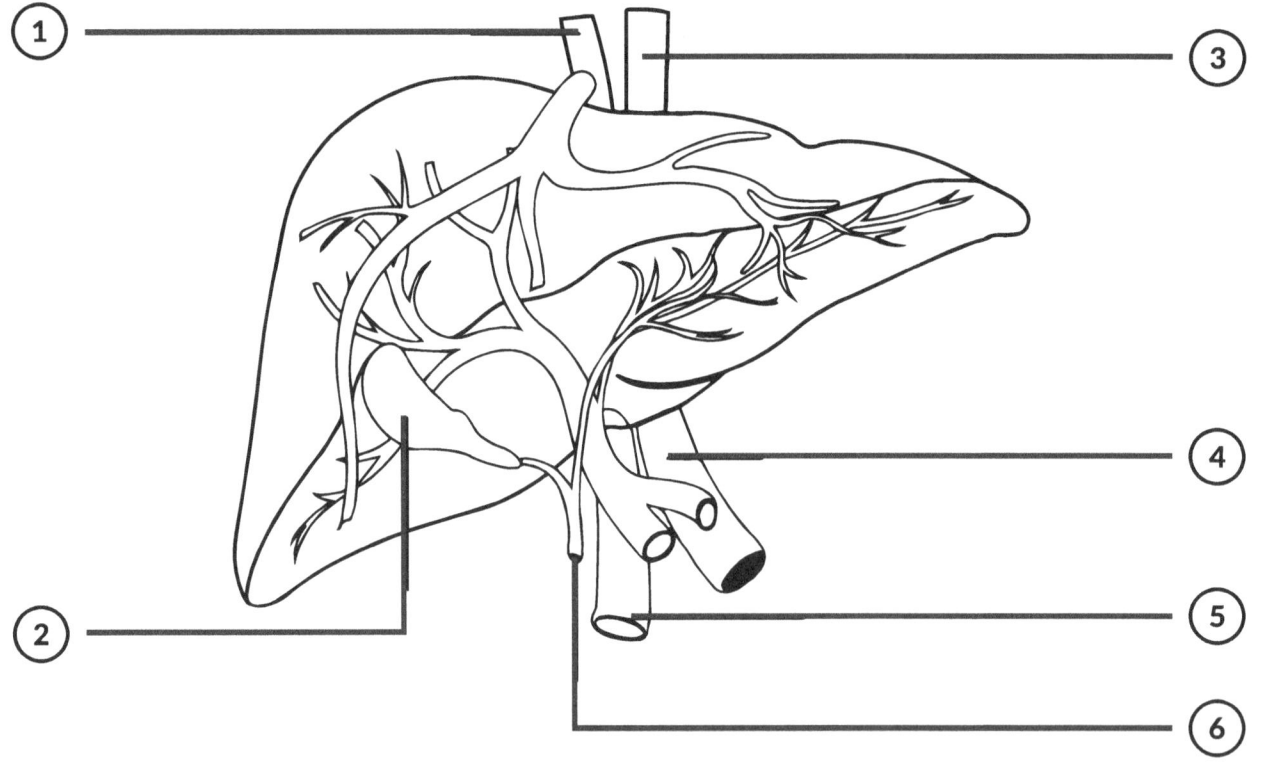

1. _____
2. _____
3. _____
4. _____
5. _____
6. _____

Liver Anatomy
(1). Inferior Vena Cava
(2). Gallbladder
(3). Aorta
(4). Hepatic Artery
(5). Portal Vein
(6). Common Bile Duct

Skin Anatomy

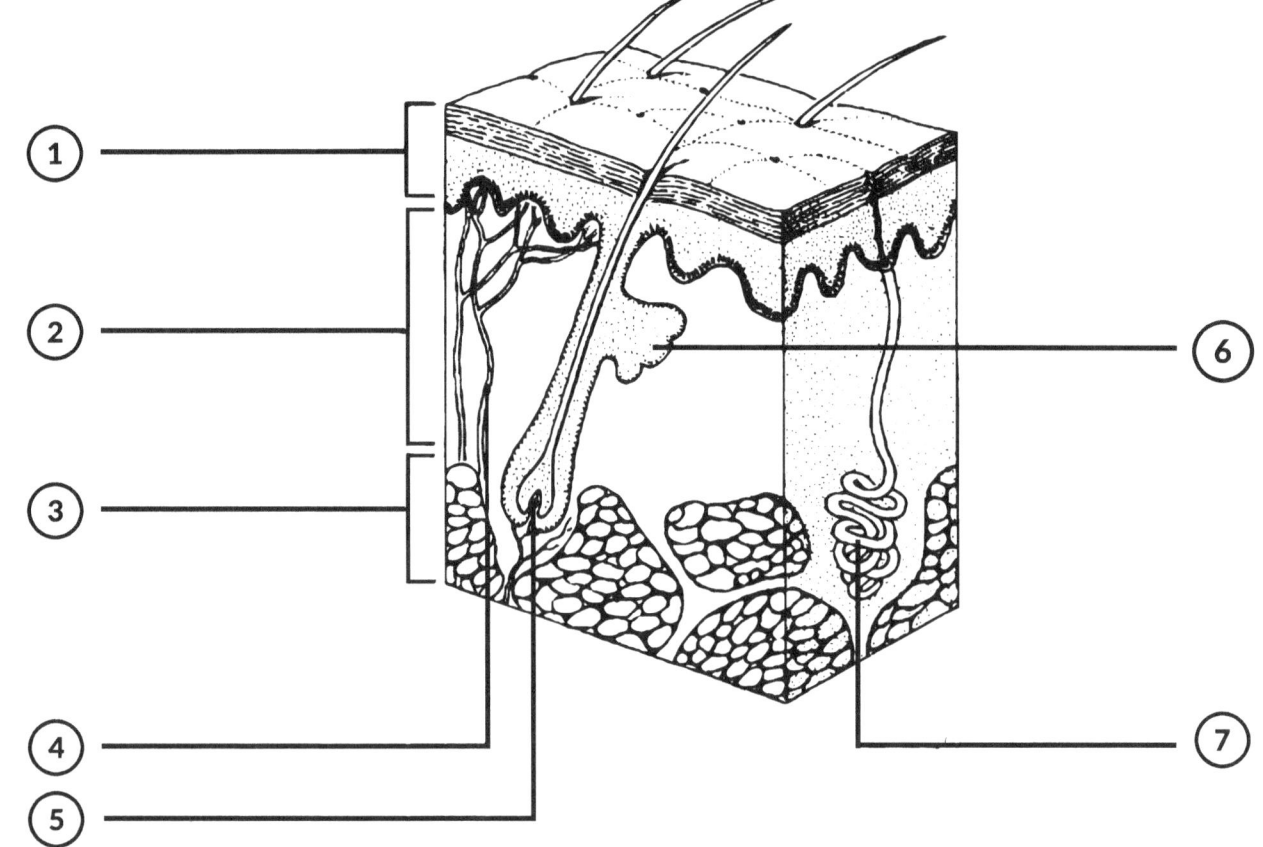

Skin Anatomy

(1). Epidermis
(2). Dermis
(3). Fatty Tissue
(4). Nerve
(5). Follicle
(6). Sweat Gland
(7). Oil Gland

Mouth and Pharynx

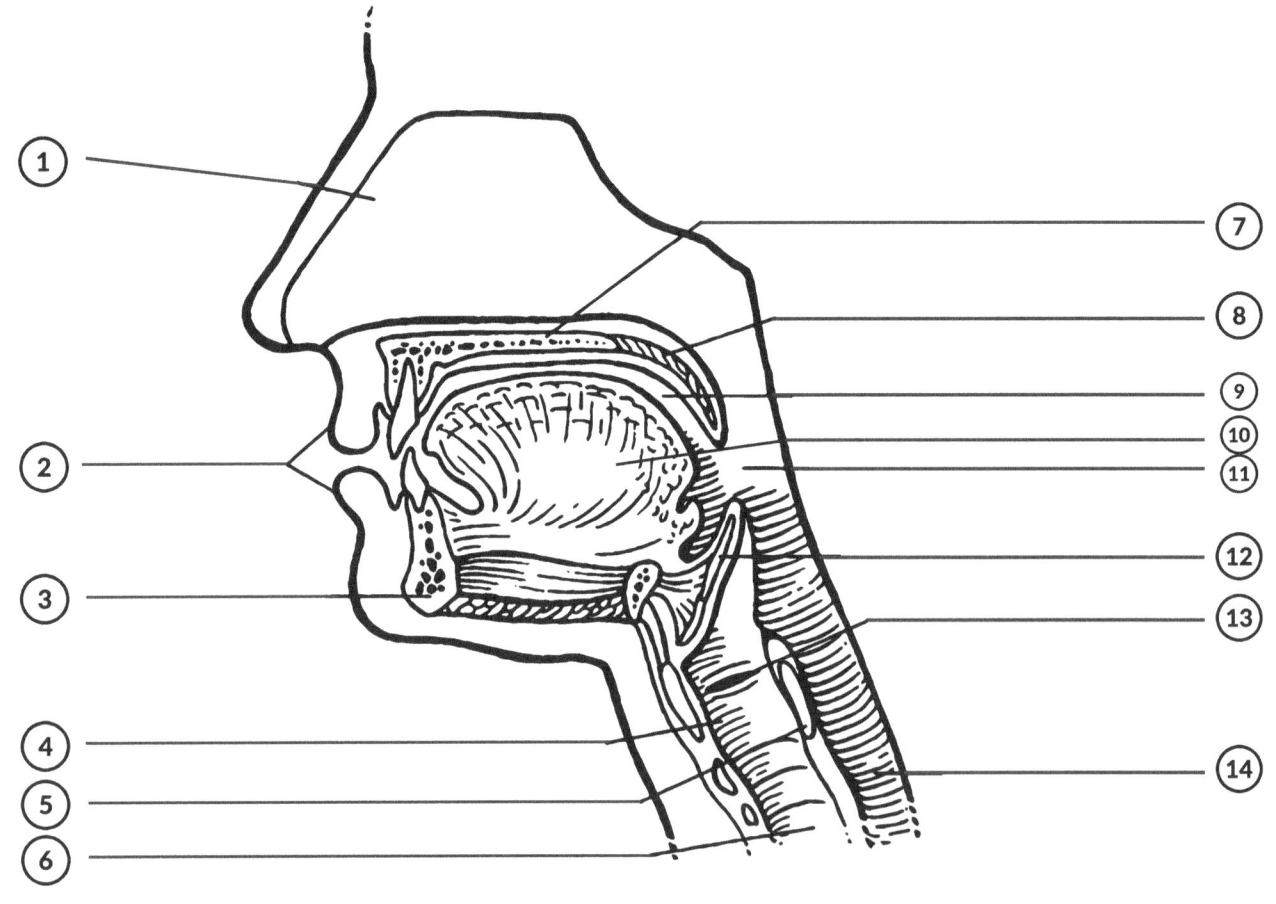

Mouth and Pharynx

(1). Nasal Cavity
(2). Lips
(3). Mandible
(4). Larynx
(5). Cricoid Cartilage
(6). Trachea (Windpipe)
(7). Hard Palate
(8). Soft Palate
(9). Oral Cavity
(10). Tongue
(11). Pharynx
(12). Epiglottis
(13). Vocal Fold
(14). Esophagus

Stomach Anatomy

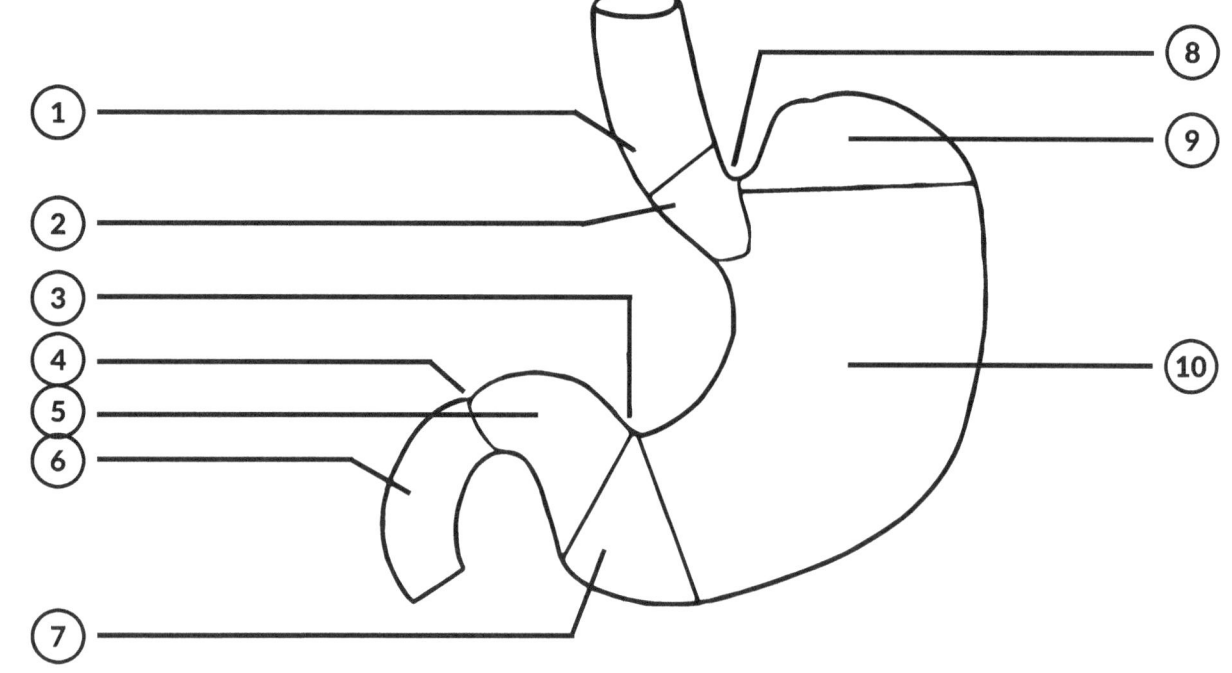

Stomach Anatomy

(1). Esophagus
(2). Cardia
(3). Angular Incisure
(4). Pylorus
(5). Pyloric Canal
(6). Duodenum
(7). Pyloric Antrum
(8). Cardiac Notch
(9). Fundus
(10). Body

Head and Neck

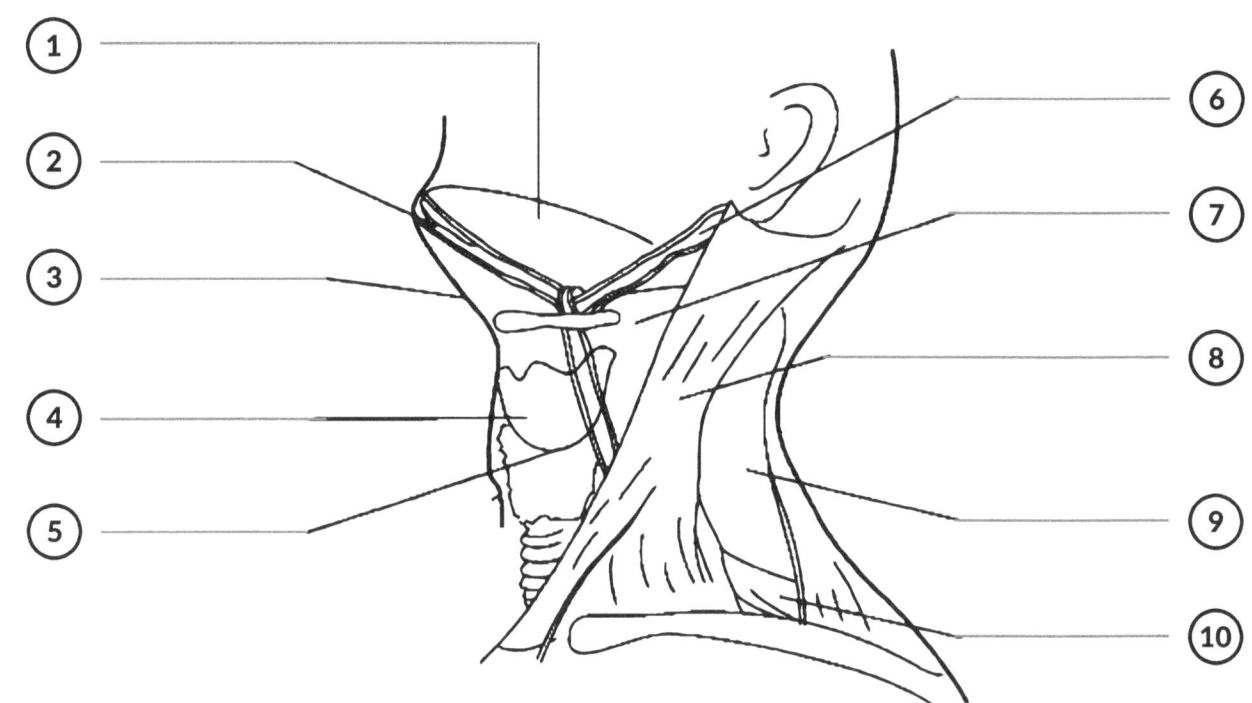

Head and Neck

(1). Submandibular Triangle
(2). Digastric Muscle
(3). Submental Triangle
(4). Muscular Triangle
(5). Omohyoid Muscle
(6). Digastric Muscle
(7). Carotid Triangle
(8). Sternocleidomastoid Muscle
(9). Lateral(Posterior)Triangle
(10). Omohyoid Muscle

Pancreas Anatomy

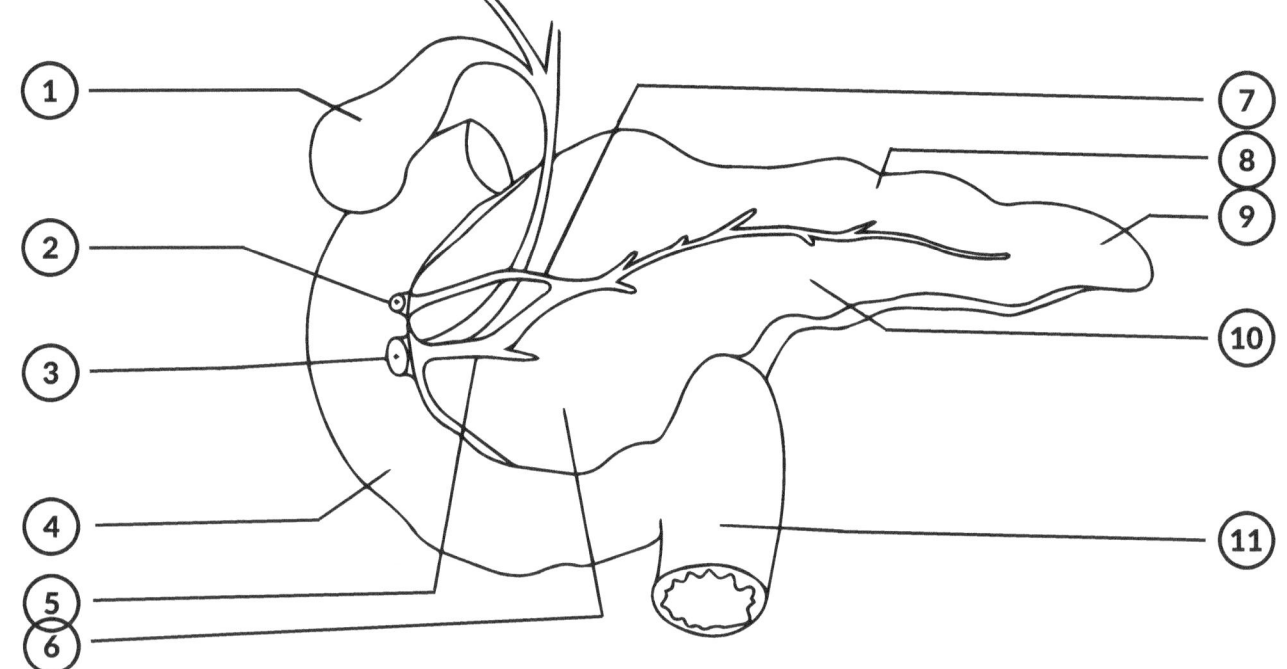

Pancreas Anatomy

(1). Gallbladder
(2). Minor Duodenal Papilla
(3). Major Duodenal Papilla
(4). Duodenum
(5). Main Pancreatic Duct
(6). Head
(7). Accessory Pancreatic Duct
(8). Pancreas
(9). Tail
(10). Body
(11). Jejunum

www.ingramcontent.com/pod-product-compliance
Lightning Source LLC
Chambersburg PA
CBHW060004230526
45472CB00008B/1946